Advanced First Aid For Survival:
When the Sh*t hits the fan <u>YOU</u> are the doctor!

Tom Sweet

Copyright © 2014 Vanguard Survival Press

All rights reserved. No part of this book may be reproduced in any manner whatsoever without express written permission except in the case of brief quotations embodied in critical articles or reviews.

DISCLAIMER

The author, Vanguard Survival, LLC, its agents, or assigns are not responsible for any misuse, injury, disability, or death that may result by the improper use of the information contained in this book. The information presented in this book is presented "As Is", without warranty to its accuracy, or applicability in any given situation or circumstance and should only be used by those with training in advanced first aid techniques. You acknowledge that your use of ANY of the information contained in this book, whether an appropriate use or not, is your SOLE RESPOSABILITY and you herby release the Author, Vanguard Survival, LLC, their agents, and assigns from all liability that may result from any misuse, injury, disability, or death.

If you are not trained in Advanced First Aid DO NOT ATTEMPT ANY OF THESE TECHNIQUES!

For information, address inquiries to:

Vanguard Survival, LLC

PO Box 893

Florissant, CO 80816

or

info@vanguardsurvival.com

First Edition 2014

ISBN: 1500535990
ISBN-13: 978-1500535995

FOREWARD

When the world goes to hell in a hand basket either because of a huge natural disaster, total collapse of society as we know it, or zombies start running around eating everything with a pulse,
YOU will become your own, or your groups, "doctor". It will be up to you to diagnose and treat various injuries and illnesses correctly to make sure that you or a member of your group "make it".

I have been in the position where I was the only person with medical training in a 500 mile radius, I was "the doctor", and I know first-hand that being able to suture a wound, place an ET tube, start an IV, or put in a chest tube has literally been the difference between life and death.

In this book I am going to cover some of the Advanced First Aid Techniques I have used and that are used by Special Operations medics to save lives every day in combat zones around the world.

Tom Sweet
Train to Survive!

CONTENTS

	Acknowledgments	i
1	A Few Words on Anatomy	1
2	Patient Assessment	Pg. 7
3	Airway Management	Pg. 18
4	Penetrating Chest Trauma	Pg. 40
5	Fluid Resuscitation	Pg.65
6	Wound Closure	Pg.85
7	Infected Wound Care	Pg.116
8	Burns	Pg.133
9	Conclusion	Pg. 152

ACKNOWLEDGMENTS

I would like to thank Dr. W. Moore, MD, Dr. W. Anderson, MD, Dr. W. Creath, DO, Dr. A. Vallena, MD, LTC J. McMillian, MD, and Dr. J. Templeton, MD for trusting me to debride wounds, place chest tubes, suture wounds, and crack a chest or two under "controlled" conditions in an ER so I would be better prepared to perform those procedures under the less controlled conditions I found myself in on occasion.
And my wife Tiffany, without your unwavering support, love, and belief in me and my dreams none of this would be possible. I thank you for all that you do to keep me motivated and focused on our goals.

1 A FEW WORDS ON ANATOMY

Before we get into the various skills and techniques used in Advanced First Aid it will help you to know some basic anatomical terms and anatomy. So before we dive into those skills and techniques I am going to toss a few $50 college words your way.

Here are a few basic anatomical terms that reference positions on the body. Knowing these terms will help you better relate the location of an injury to emergency personnel should the need arise. To do so you have to divide the body with a series of imaginary lines called planes.

Planes of the Body

A plane is a surface in which if any two points are taken, a straight line that is drawn to join these two points lies wholly within that plane or surface. The planes of the body are:
- Medial Plane- A vertical plane running from front to back (Anterior-Posterior) dividing the body into right and left parts. The plane divides the body into equal right and left parts by running through the middle of the breast bone (sternum).
- Medial Plane of an Extremity- A plane running lengthwise through an extremity from front to back. This plane must pass through the third finger of the hand or second toe of the foot. It is used as a reference plane to movements that involve spreading the toes or fingers (except thumb) apart or together. moving them together.
- Transverse Plane- A plane that divides the body or limbs into upper and lower parts in relation to gravity and anatomical position.

- Frontal Plane- A plane dividing the body into Anterior (front) and posterior (back) portions.

Anatomical Position Terms

- Anterior-Refers to the front of the body
- Posterior- Refers to the back of the body
- Medial Line-Refers to an imaginary line that runs right through the center of the body from the head to the feet
- Lateral-Refers to a point or area that is more distant from the medial plane. The outer side of the elbow is lateral when compared with for example, the inner side.
- Superior-Towards the head
- Inferior-Towards the feet
- Proximal-Nearest; closer to any point of reference. An example is the elbow is proximal to the wrist on the upper extremity
- Distal- Remote; farther from any point of reference. An example is the elbow is distal to the shoulder joint.

Below is a diagram of the relative anatomical positions.

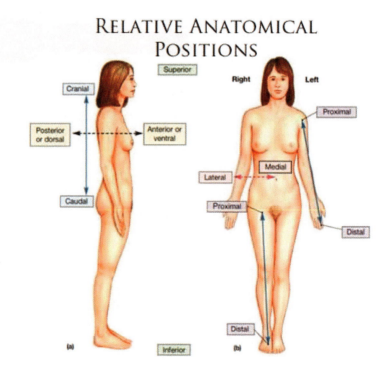

Skeletal Anatomy

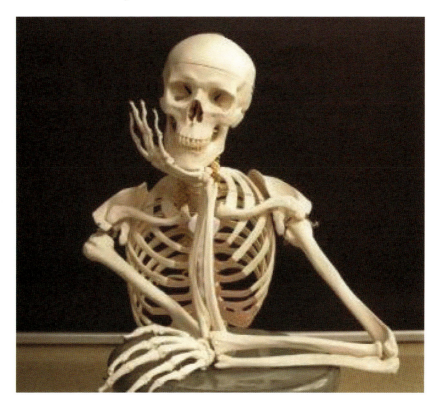

The human skeleton is lighter than stainless steel, as tough as reinforced concrete, and able to repair itself. The skeletal system is the scaffolding that allows you to walk upright, the various bones, ligaments, and tendons protect your internal organs and allow you to move. Without the skeleton we'd all just be a big pile of mushy flesh. I won't go into every single ligament and tendon since those are beyond the scope of this book but, It helps to know what bones are where in order to better understand why something doesn't function like it is supposed to in the event of an injury. There are 102 bones in the human body and each has a specific function in protecting organs and allowing you to move.

On the next page you will see a diagram that shows the skeletal anatomy and its many pieces.

Diagram of skeletal anatomy

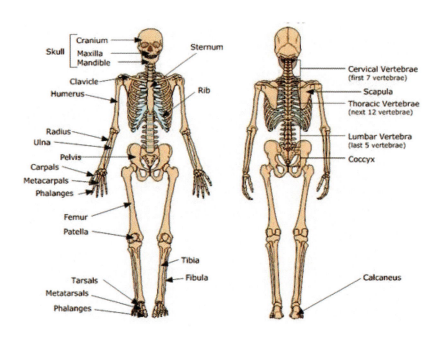

Circulatory System

The circulatory system consists of the heart, blood, veins and arteries and is a "closed system" (or at least it is supposed to be). The heart pumps approximately 5 liters of blood throughout the body, using the system of arteries and veins, transporting oxygenated blood and nutrients throughout the body per minute.

The average heartbeat is 72 times per minute. In the course of one day it beats over 100,000 times. In one year the heart beats almost 38 million times, and by the time you are 70 years old, on average, it beats 2.5 billion times!

Average Pulse Rates By Age

Newborn   130
3 months   140
6 months   130
1 year   120
2 years   115
3 years   100
4 years   100
6 years   100
8 years   90
12 years   85
Adult   60 - 100

By having a basic understanding of the circulatory system you will be better equipped to treat any disruption to that system to stop bleeding that can lead to life threatening complications. Below is a simple diagram of the human circulatory system.

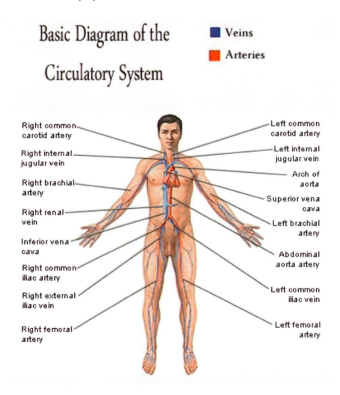

Tom Sweet

2 PATIENT ASSESSMENT

Now that you have a little better understanding of the human body and its various "systems" before you can treat any injury or illness you first have to find it. By doing a patient assessment you can do just that, find the problem and correct it.

Primary Survey

The standard "ABC" approach as outlined in PHTLS (Pre-Hospital Trauma Life Support), ATLS (Advanced Trauma Life Support), and AHA (American Heart Association) CPR guidelines provides an excellent method for addressing life-threatening injuries in a systematic fashion.

The "ABC" pneumonic prioritizes the search for injuries in accordance with their potential to kill the patient; it is simple to remember and it provides an anchor point from which patients can re-assessed if they deteriorate.

This system may require some modification in a survival or SHTF setting.

For example, in a survival or SHTF situation where you have mass casualties, you may need to address the "ABCs" of several patients at once. Simply asking them where they are injured can do this. Those casualties who answer the question appropriately have an intact airway, are breathing and are conscious.

You should then focus his attention on those casualties who are unconscious or in obvious distress. Meanwhile, you can direct the lightly injured casualties or non-medical members of your group to aid in controlling the bleeding of those patients with active hemorrhage, thus addressing the circulation step.

During a SHTF situation where you are taking fire, moving the patient to a safe location takes priority over the Primary and Secondary Survey unless a rapid maneuver can be performed for an obvious life-threatening injury, i.e., the application of a tourniquet. Rapid control of hemorrhage is a mainstay of this type of casualty care.

Airway

A conscious spontaneously breathing patient requires no immediate airway intervention. If the patient is able to talk normally his airway is intact. If the patient is semi-conscious or unconscious, the flaccid tongue is the most common source of airway obstruction. The chin lift or jaw thrust maneuver should be attempted and should readily relieve any obstruction created by the tongue.

Once the airway is opened or if further difficulty is encountered, a nasopharyngeal or oropharyngeal airway should be inserted. The nasopharyngeal airway is better tolerated in the semi-conscious patient and the patient with an intact gag reflex.

If the above measures fail to provide an adequate airway or if the patient is unconscious, unresponsive and apneic, orotracheal intubation should be considered. Orotracheal intubation done on a trauma patient with an intact gag reflex without the use of pharmacological sedation and paralysis will be difficult and may cause additional complications such as vomiting, airway trauma and increased intracranial pressure, and thus should be avoided except as a last resort.

If the patient is breathing and definitive airway control if needed, blind nasotracheal intubation (BNTI) may be attempted. Severe facial fractures and basilar skull fractures are relative contraindications to BNTI.

Other adjuncts to airway management can and should be used if available and if your are skilled in their use. Other possible adjuncts to airway management include the Laryngeal Mask Airway (LMA) the Intubating LMA, the Combitube, and the Lighted Stylet.

If the patient has obvious face, mouth, or jaw trauma with signs of airway compromise or if orotracheal intubation fails, then a surgical cricothyroidotomy may be a necessary and lifesaving maneuver, which we will cover a little later.

The most common mistake when performing a surgical airway is delaying too long before starting the procedure. Civilian models of trauma care include cervical spine control and immobilization with airway management.

Few if any casualties with penetrating trauma will have associated injury to the cervical spine (based on surveys done in Iraq and Afghanistan of combat casualties) unless they have combined blunt injuries from vehicle or aircraft crashes, falls or crush injuries, or penetrating injury to the spinal cord.

Meticulous attention to presumed cervical spine injury in a survival or SHTF situation is not warranted if penetrating trauma is the obvious injury. Furthermore, you or the casualty may sustain additional injury if treatment of other injuries such as bleeding is delayed while the cervical spine is immobilized.

Breathing

In the conscious patient, who is alert and breathing normally, no interventions are required. If the patient has signs of respiratory distress such as tachypnea (very rapid breathing), dyspnea (difficulty breathing), or cyanosis (bluish coloration of the lips or skin), which may be associated with agitation or decreasing mental status, an aggressive search for why is required.

Injuries that may result in significant respiratory compromise include tension pneumothorax, open pneumothorax (sucking chest wound), flail chest, and massive hemothorax. The patient's chest and back should be quickly exposed and inspected for obvious signs of trauma, asymmetrical or paradoxical movement of the chest wall, accessory muscle use and jugular venous distention (obvious swelling in the jugular vein(s)).

If possible, auscultation (listening) should be performed listening for abnormal or decreased breath sounds. The chest wall should be palpated to identify areas of tenderness, crepitus, subcutaneous emphysema or deformity.

Open pneumothorax should be treated with a three-sided occlusive dressing and a tension pneumothorax with needle decompression, which we will cover a little later.

The field management of a flail chest centers on controlling the patient's pain and augmentation of the patient's respiratory efforts with bag valve mask ventilation.

Chest wall splinting with tape, sandbags and the like has been advocated in the past but should no longer be performed as it decreases the movement of the chest wall and will further compromise the patient's ability to ventilate. These casualties may have significant injury to the underlying lung and may deteriorate rapidly requiring endotracheal intubation and positive pressure ventilation.

Management of a massive hemothorax in the field should be directed at maintaining adequate ventilation with a BVM. If rescue is delayed and the patient continues to deteriorate, consideration may be given for the placement of a chest tube, which will be covered later. If more than 1000cc of blood is immediately drained by the chest tube or if the output is more than 200cc per hour for 4 hours, the patient likely has injury to the great vessels, hilum, heart or vessels in the chest wall that will require surgical repair. Flail chest and massive hemothorax are difficult injuries to treat in the field and should be evacuated are rapidly as possible.

Circulation

Next to environmental causes (hypothermia and hyperthermia) uncontrolled bleeding is the leading cause of preventable deaths in a survival or SHTF situations. Rapid identification and effective management of bleeding is perhaps the single most important aspect of the primary survey while caring for a casualty in a survival or SHTF situation.

Obvious external sources of bleeding should be controlled with direct pressure initially followed by a field dressing or pressure dressing. If bleeding is not controlled by the previous measures or if gross arterial bleeding is present, an effective tourniquet should immediately be applied.

Clamping of injured vessels is not indicated unless the bleeding vessel can be directly visualized. Blind clamping of vessels may result in additional injury to neurovascular structures and should not be done.

NOTE: The current ATLS manual discourages the use of tourniquets in the pre-hospital setting because of distal tissue ischemia, tissue crush injury at the tourniquet site, which may necessitate subsequent amputation.

This admonition is based on a model of trauma care where most penetrating injuries are low velocity in nature and rapid evacuation to a trauma center is available. Withholding the use of tourniquets in a survival or SHTF situation for patients with severe extremity bleeding may result in death or injury that might have otherwise been prevented.

Sources of internal bleeding should be identified. A significant amount of blood can be lost into the chest and abdominal cavities, the retroperitoneal space and the soft tissues surrounding fractures of the pelvis and lower extremities.

Significant bleeding into the thoracic and abdominal cavities following trauma will require surgical exploration. In the absence of a head injury, hypotensive (low blood pressure) resuscitation will help prevent more bleeding.

Bleeding from injuries to the pelvis and groin or from fractures of the lower extremities not otherwise amenable to treatment with a tourniquet and not associated with thoracic injuries may be controlled with the application of Pneumatic Anti-Shock Garment (PASG), AKA Military Anti-Shock Trousers (MAST), which you can find for sale on eBay from time to time.

After sources of hemorrhage are identified and controlled, the need for intravenous access, which we will cover later, should be considered. If the patient has an isolated extremity wound, the bleeding has been controlled and there are no signs of shock, there is no need for immediate intravenous fluid resuscitation.

Intravenous access with a saline lock should be considered for all casualties with significant injuries. If there is a truncal injury and if signs of shock are present, or if blood pressure continues to drop, intravenous access should be obtained with a 12 to 16-gauge catheter followed by a 1-2 liter bolus of normal saline or lactated Ringers, or 500 milliliters of Hespan.

If the patient has improvement of the clinical signs of shock following the initial bolus, subsequent intravenous fluids should be given to achieve only a good peripheral pulse and an improvement in sensorium rather than to normalize blood pressure.

If there is no clinical improvement following the initial IV fluid bolus, the possibility of severe uncontrolled intra-abdominal or intrathoracic bleeding should be considered.

Further fluid resuscitation in uncontrolled hemorrhage is not indicated, may be harmful, and may waste the limited fluids available in a survival or

SHTF situation.

Cardiopulmonary arrest from hemorrhage has a very high mortality in the hospital setting. Attempting to resuscitate patients who are in cardiac arrest secondary to hemorrhage while in the field will almost certainly be futile.

Disability

A brief neurological assessment should be performed using the AVPU scale:
- A-Alert
- V-Responds to verbal stimuli; you ask a question, the patient answers
- P- Responds to painful stimuli; the patient responds to a pinch on the arm or sternal rub
- U-Unresponsive; the patient does not respond to any form of stimuli

After you have determined the patients neurological status using AVPU you want to determine if they are oriented to time, person, and place. Asking questions like, "Who is the president?" "What day of the week is it?" "Where are you?" Do you know what happened?" What's your name?" and my personal favorite while I was a medic, "Is Mickey Mouse a cat or a dog?"

By asking these questions you can determine very quickly the mental status of your patient. Suspect some type of head injury in anyone who can't answer these basic questions.

Exposure

Clothing and protective equipment such as and body armor should only be removed as required to evaluate and treat specific injuries. If the patient is conscious with a single extremity injury or wound, only the area surrounding the injury should be exposed.

Unconscious patients may require more extensive exposure in order to discover potentially serious injuries but must subsequently be protected from the elements and the environment. Hypothermia is to be avoided in trauma patients at all costs.

Vital Signs

Vital signs should be assessed frequently, especially after specific therapeutic interventions (IV's, Airway placement, etc.), and before and after moving patients. You should be sensitive to subtle changes in vital signs in wounded or injured members of your group.

Be aware that someone in great physical shape may have a greater reserve and ability to compensate for blood loss longer than someone who is not in as good of physical shape and therefore they may not manifest significant changes in vital signs until they are in severe shock.

The vital signs include:

- **Pulse:** The rate and character of the pulse should be evaluated. A weak, rapid, barely palpable (felt) radial pulse indicates the presence of hemorrhagic shock.
- **Respiration:** Respiratory rate can be an extremely sensitive indicator of physiologic stress. Resting tachypnea (rapid breathing) should be considered abnormal and should prompt investigation if there is no obvious cause.
- **Blood Pressure:** You aren't going to be expected to carry a Blood Pressure Cuff in your medical bag or survival kit. But palpation of distal and central pulses provides a rough guide to systolic blood pressure.
- **Radial**- at least 70 mmHg
- **Femoral**- at least 60 mmHg
- **Carotid**- at least 50 mmHg

Temperature: Only if hypo or hyperthermia are suspected. Hypothermia is an often unrecognized and yet significant contributor to traumatic death.

Secondary Survey

After you have found and treated the immediate, life threatening injuries or conditions you found in the Primary Survey it is time to conduct a Secondary Survey.

The Secondary Survey, is a more methodical search for non-life threatening injuries. These injuries should be treated as they are encountered. Like the Primary Survey above, the Secondary Survey may need to be modified and adapted according to the tactical situation and the number and type of casualties encountered.

The vast majority (75%) of casualties in a survival or SHTF situation will have isolated penetrating trauma to the extremities. These patients do not require a detailed head to toe exam in the Secondary Survey.

They will need to have a bandage and/or splint applied with evaluation of their neurovascular status distal to the injury before and after treatment. They then need to be frequently reassessed for signs of deterioration as the situation permits.

Patients who are severely injured or unconscious will require a more detailed Secondary Survey as outlined below. Evacuation from a hostile area or situation should not be delayed to perform a Secondary Survey or for the treatment of non-life threatening injuries.

The Secondary Survey should be conducted in a systematic head to toe, front to back fashion using visual Inspection, Auscultation, and Palpation (IAP) where applicable. In children the Secondary Survey should be conducted in a Toe to Head fashion to alleviate fear and put the child at ease.

HEENT (Head, Ears, Eyes, Nose, Throat)

The head and face should be inspected for obvious laceration, burns, contusion, asymmetry or hemorrhage.

The bones of the face and head should then be palpated to identify crepitus, bony step-off, depressions or abnormal mobility of the mandible and mid-face.

The eyes should be opened and examined for signs of trauma, globe rupture, or hyphema. The orbits and zygomatic arches should be palpated for signs of fractures. Pupils should be checked for reactivity and symmetry. If the patient is awake, extra-ocular movements can be assessed along with gross visual acuity.

The ears should be inspected for obvious trauma and the ear canals for blood or cerebrospinal fluid (CSF). Battle's sign indicating possible basilar skull fracture may be observed over the mastoid processes. The nares should be inspected for blood or CSF.

The mouth and oropharynx should be inspected for trauma or bleeding. Loose teeth, dental appliances or other potential airway obstructions should be removed. Any previous airway interventions should be reassessed.

Neck

The neck should be visually inspected searching for obvious trauma or deformity, tracheal deviation, jugular venous distention (JVD), or signs of respiratory accessory muscle use. The cervical spine should be palpated for step-off, tenderness or deformity.

Chest

The chest wall should be observed for penetrating injury or blunt injury, asymmetrical breathing movements (only one side of the chest moves when the patient breathes or one side rises and the other falls) or retractions (pulling inward of the muscles surrounding the rib cage).

Auscultation over the anterior lung fields, posterior lung bases and heart should follow. The entire rib cage, sternum and chest wall should be palpated for tenderness, flail segments, subcutaneous
emphysema (Air under and in the skin) or crepitus (bonne grating on bone). Percussion may be performed looking for hyper-resonance or dullness.

Abdomen

The abdomen should be observed for signs of blunt or penetrating injury. The presence or absence of bowel sounds should evaluated. Palpation searching for tenderness, guarding or rigidity should
follow. Percussion may elicit subtle rebound tenderness.

Pelvis

The pelvis should be inspected for signs of penetrating trauma or deformity. Pelvic instability and fracture should be suspected with movement of the anterior iliac crests when lateral and anterior pressure is applied.

The perineum and genitals are inspected next for signs of injury. Scrotal, vulvar and perineal hematomas or blood at the urethral meatus may indicate pelvic fracture.

Extremities

The extremities are inspected and palpated proximally to distally. Each bone and joint distal to the pelvis and clavicle should be assessed for crepitus, tenderness, deformity and abnormal joint motion.

Distal pulses and capillary refill are then examined. Asking the patient if he can feel the examiner lightly touching his hands and feet tests gross sensation.

Gross motor strength is tested by having the patient squeeze the examiner's fingers and by moving his toes up and down against the resistance of the examiner's hands.

Neurological

A field neurological exam should consist of observation of the pupils for reactivity and asymmetry (done during HEENT exam), the level of consciousness, gross sensory and motor function (assessed during examination of the extremities) and calculation of the Glasgow Coma Scale (GCS).

Glasgow Coma Scale

Eye Opening

Spontaneous	4
Verbal	3
Pain	2
No Response	1

Best Verbal Response

Oriented	4
Confused	3
Inappropriate Words	2
None	1

Best Motor Response

Obeys Commands   6

Localizes Pain   5

Withdraws from Pain 4

Flexion   3

Extension   2

None   1

Total 3-15

Any patient with a GCS of 8 or less is considered to have a severe head injury. Those in the 9 to 12 range are considered moderate, but may require airway control. Any GCS of 13 to 15 is considered indicative of mild or no head injury, but even these patients can deteriorate and should be observed.

The GCS is a useful tool that can be used to monitor the clinical status of seriously injured patients. A declining GCS score over time indicates further neurological deterioration. A GCS less than 9 indicates severe neurological injury. A GCS of less than 8, intubate if you are able to, if not you have to ensure and maintain an airway since these patient more than likely can't maintain one themselves.

Now that you have a better understanding of human anatomy and the initial steps you need to take to treat injuries sustained in a survival or SHTF situation you will better able to recognize when a particular intervention or technique is needed.

3 AIRWAY MANAGEMENT

Making sure your patient has a patent (open) airway is the first thing you need to do no matter what injury or illness they may have. Without an open airway they won't be doing a whole lot of that in and out, in and out, breathing thing that we all need in order to survive.

In this chapter we are going to cover some ways that you can maintain and control your patents airway and make sure they keep doing that in and out breathing thing.

Basic Airway Management

The first thing you can do to check for an open airway is simply talk to your patient. Ask simple questions and if the patient can answer you without any difficulty they have an open airway. Pretty simple, huh?

If your patient can't answer questions or you see obvious signs of distress you can use the Head Tilt, Chin Lift, or if you suspect any kind of neck injury, the Jaw Thrust. Both of these techniques open the airway by moving the most common cause of airway obstruction, the tongue.

Check the diagrams on the next page for how to perform the Head Tilt, Chin Lift and Jaw Thrust.

The Head Tilt, Chin Lift method of opening the airway.

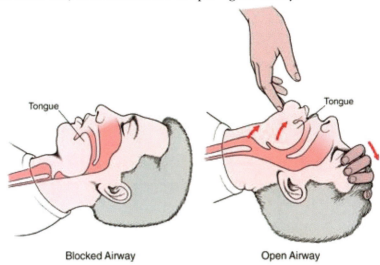

The Jaw Thrust method of opening the airway.

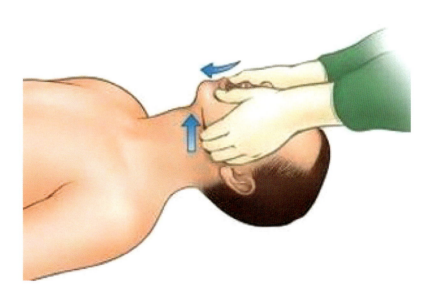

In a patient who is conscious and has an intact gag reflex but needs some help maintaining an airway you can use a **nasopharyngeal** airway (NPA). The correct airway should go from the patients nose to their earlobe, if it goes past their earlobe it is too long and if it doesn't touch their earlobe it is too short, either situation can be bad for your patient so make sure you have the right airway for the patient you are treating.

The photo below shows the correct way to measure a nasal airway.

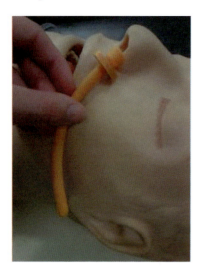

Once you have the correct size airway that little package of lubricant you should have does help these things go in faster and it reduces damage to the nasal mucosa but don't waste too much time coating the NPA with a shiny sheen of lube. Tear open the packet, squirt a clump of lube on the lower half of the NPA and get on with it.

It doesn't need a full, even, double coat of lubrication Bob Vila, and it doesn't need a Swedish massage either. It needs to get sunk it the nasal passage and you need to get on with managing the airway.

If you took an EMT class they probably made a big deal about placing the bevel toward the septum. That is the preferred insertion technique, but nobody has ever really been able to convincingly explain to me why that is nor have I ever stuck to it like gospel.

Note that most NPAs are designed to be inserted in the right nostril. (If you follow the bevel rule.) But we also tell you to pick the largest nare. So which takes precedence? Should we never use the left nare regardless of how tiny the right one might look? Or perhaps insert the NPA backwards?

Do neither. Insert it in the largest nare with the curve of the NPA oriented toward the mouth and forget about the bevel.

Some folks will tell you to wiggle that thing back and forth like you're trying to start a fire or something. Take it easy boy scout.

Yes we want you to use a gentle back and forth motion on the NPA as you insert it, but you don't need to over-do it. Once you reach the mid-point of the NPA you should be able to just sink it.

And your patient will thank you for it later. The wiggling may facilitate the advance of the device but it isn't terribly comfortable on the patients nose.

For the record these things aren't going up the patient's nose. They go straight back in to the nasal cavity and turn downward toward the posterior pharynx.

A patient I worked on in Iraq with a nasal airway in place.

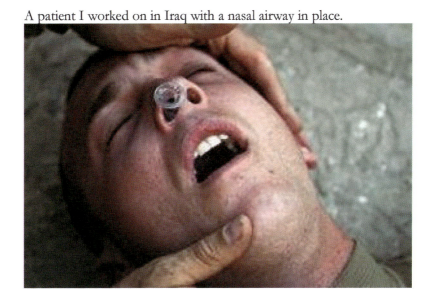

For patients who are unconscious or those who don't have a gag reflex you can use an oral airway. Like the nasal airway you have to measure it first. You do this by placing the large flange of the airway at the corner of the mouth and measure to the earlobe again. If it goes past the earlobe it is too big and if it doesn't touch the earlobe it is too same.

The picture below shows how to measure an oral airway.

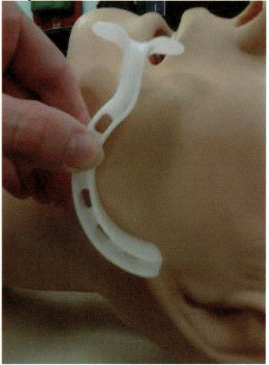

Remove any dentures, loose or broken teeth, or any other removable dental appliance. Once you are sure there is nothing in the patients mouth it is time to place the airway.

First, open the patient's mouth using the cross-finger method, placing your thumb on the patient's bottom teeth and your index finger on the upper teeth, then gently pushing them apart. With the patient's mouth open as wide as possible, begin inserting the airway upside down (hook up), with the curvature toward the tongue to prevent pushing the tongue back into the pharynx.

Avoid dislodging teeth or damaging mouth tissue by gently sliding the airway over the tongue toward the back of the mouth. When the airway reaches the back of the tongue, rotate the device 180 degrees.

The tip should point down as it approaches the posterior wall of the pharynx, and the curvature should follow the contour of the roof of the mouth.

An alternative method is to hold the airway in its normal upright position and use a tongue depressor to hold the tongue down. Slide the airway carefully over the tongue and into position.

If the patient gags or appears to be gasping for air after insertion, remove the airway immediately. Recheck the size before attempting reinsertion.

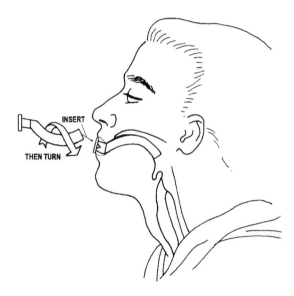

Advanced Airway Management

When basic airway management techniques aren't enough or a longer term solution is needed there are a few advanced airway management techniques you can use to ensure that your patient has a good secured airway.

Endotracheal Intubation

First, evaluate the airway during the initial injury assessment, and administer supplemental oxygen during this time if possible. Continual airway assessment is crucial since subtle changes in mental or respiratory status can occur at any time. Airway characteristics that can make fitting the mask and endotracheal intubation difficult include:

- Short, thick, muscular or fat neck with full set of teeth;
- Full beard, facial burns, or facial injuries;
- Receding or malformed jaw;
- Protruding maxillary incisors; and
- Poor mandibular (lower jaw) mobility.

Co-existing injuries such as known or suspected cervical spine injury, thoracic trauma, skull fractures, scalp lacerations, ocular injuries and airway trauma must be included when planning airway management.

Indications for endotracheal intubation include anatomic traits making airway management with just a mask difficult or impossible, the need for frequent suctioning, prevention of aspiration of gastric contents, respiratory failure or insufficiency, disease or trauma to airway, and traumatic injuries or musculoskeletal malformations making ventilation difficult.

Whenever possible O2 should be used when you intubate a patient, obviously this may not be possible in a survival or SHTF situation so at the very least you should have an appropriate sized Bag-Valve-Mask (BVM) available to provide proper ventilation to the patient while they are intubated.

The list below shows the average ET tube and Laryngoscope blade size to use by age.

Endotracheal tube and Laryngoscope Blade sizes:

Age:	Preemie	Neonate	6 mo.	1-2 yr.	4-6 yr.	8-12 yr.	Adult
Tube size:	2.5	3-3.5	3.5-4	4-5	5-5.5	6-7	7.5-8.5
Blade size:	0	0-1	1	1-2	2	2-3	4-5

The picture below shows the equipment needed to perform ET tube or other airway placement.

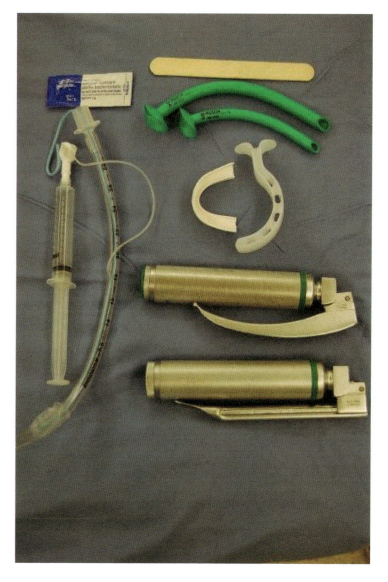

The following pictures show you the proper blade placement to intubate your patient.

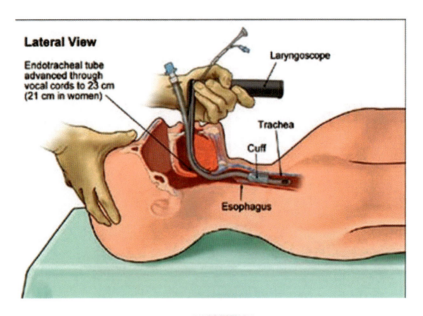

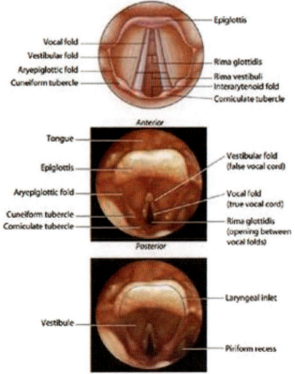

Superior view through the laryngeal inlet

Use the following steps to intubate your patient.

1. Gather and check all equipment for proper function. Check light on laryngoscope, inflate ET cuff with 5-10cc air and check for leaks, then deflate and leave syringe attached, you can insert a lubricated stylet so it does not protrude beyond distal end of ET tube and bend into hockey stick form, and have suction on, if available.

2. Hyperventilate with 100% O2 for several minutes using BVM, if available.

3. Have assistant hold cricoid pressure if aspiration is a risk.

4. If orotracheal intubation is planned, hold the laryngoscope in left hand and insert the blade on right side of mouth pushing the tongue to the left in a sweeping motion, and avoiding the lips, teeth and tongue. Holding the left wrist rigid, to avoid using the scope as a fulcrum and damaging the teeth, visualize the epiglottis.

5. If a straight (Miller) blade is used, pass the blade tip beneath the laryngeal surface of the epiglottis and lift forward and upward to expose the glottic opening.

6. If a curved (Macintosh) blade is used, advance the tip of the blade into the space between the base of the tongue and the pharyngeal surface of the epiglottis (the vallecula) to expose the glottic opening.

7. Insert the ET with the right hand through the vocal cords until the cuff disappears.

8. Remove the stylet and advance the tube slightly further. Inflate the cuff with air until no leak is heard when ventilated with bag.

9. Usually, adult women use a 6.5 to 7.0mm; men use a 7.5 to 8.0mm ET tube.

10. Verify correct placement by listening over both lungs for bilateral, equal breath sounds and observe the chest for symmetric, bilateral movements.

11. Listen over the stomach, where you should not hear breath sounds.

12. Note depth of insertion by centimeter markings on the tube at the lips, and tape the tube in place.

Nasotracheal Intubation

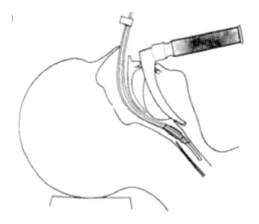

When the mouth cannot be opened or the patient cannot be ventilated by another means, or if the patient is conscious and requiring intubation, follow steps 1-3 for Orotracheal intubation using a lubricated (water-soluble), size 7-7.5 ET without the stylet.

1. Insert the ET tube straight down into the larger of the nostrils until it reaches the posterior pharyngeal wall.

2. If doing a blind nasal intubation, listen for the patient to inhale and insert the ET quickly into the trachea with a single smooth motion.

3. If intubating under direct visualization, now insert the blade as previously described and pass the ET through the cords.

4. Inflate the cuff and verify placement as above.

Combitube

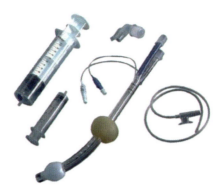

The Combitube is almost an ideal rescue airway. The availability of a Combitube makes rapid sequence intubation a safe procedure. The standard size will function well in almost any adult. The smaller size is available for persons between 4- and 5-feet tall. Many Asian and Hispanic patients may be less than 5-feet tall. The volume of air in the large balloon is reduced to 80 cc in the 4-feet tall model.

The esophageal tracheal Combitube (Combitube™) is a two-barreled tube that functions well when placed in either the trachea or the esophagus. Insertion does not require neck movement. *Note: The short white tube is connected to the end of the tube; the long blue tube is connected to the side holes located between the two balloons.*

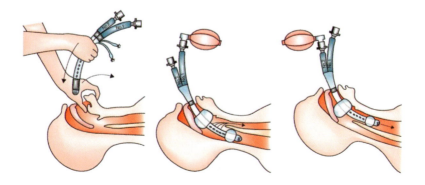

1. The tube is placed blindly with care to keep it midline. It is placed

to a depth that lines up the teeth between the 2 proximal markings on the tube. Placing the tube too deeply will occlude the larynx.

2. The large 100 cc balloon is inflated in the posterior pharynx; the 15 cc distal balloon is then inflated. While the large cuff is inflating, it will want to move the Combitube in or out. It is conforming to the posterior pharynx and palate. Let it move.

3. The short white tube is continuous with the distal opening of the tube. Attach an esophageal intubation detector (EID) and test it for position. Do it twice if the patient has been bag-valve-mask ventilated. Alternatively, simply begin ventilation through the long blue tube and observe for chest rise and listen for breath sounds. About 90% of the time, the Combitube will be in the esophagus. If the tube does not function, it is probably in the trachea.

4. If the tube is in the trachea, use it like an endotracheal tube. Ventilate through the short white tube. The large balloon stabilizes the Combitube and keeps it in correct position.

If the Combitube is functioning well, there is no need to replace it during resuscitation or for transfer. However, to avoid error, bend the unused tube down and tape it there.

To replace the Combitube with a regular ET tube when it is located in the trachea, pass an ET tube introducer (ETI) through the white tube and remove the Combitube. Pass a regular ET tube into the trachea over the ETI.

It the Combitube is in the esophagus, and you wish to replace it with an ET tube, the trachea can be intubated with difficulty without removing the tube. Deflate the large balloon and move the tube to the side of the mouth. Use a laryngoscope to visualize the larynx by lifting the base of the tongue. The deflated large balloon can still obstruct your vision. If this occurs, rotate the Combitube to change the orientation of the deflated balloon. Intubate with the aid of an ETI.

Alternatively, pass a lubricated 14 French gastric tube through the white tube to evacuate the esophagus and stomach. Deflate both balloons, remove the esophageal tracheal Combitube, and intubate as usual.

If the patient is conscious, the Combitube is uncomfortable. Sedation is needed. A Combitube is not adequate to ventilate a patient with laryngospasm unless paralysis is used. Laryngeal edema is a relative contraindication. The latex balloon may be a problem in latex-sensitive individuals.

The Combitube is not suitable for use over a long period (over about 2 to 3 hours). The Combitube offers slight resistance to exhalation when placed in the esophagus.

Needle and Surgical Cricothyroidotomy

Needle cricothyroidotomy involves passing an over-the-needle IV catheter through the cricothyroid membrane. This procedure provides a temporary secure airway to oxygenate and ventilate a patient in severe respiratory distress in whom less invasive techniques (e.g., bag-valve-mask ventilation, laryngeal mask ventilation, endotracheal intubation) have failed or are not likely to be successful (i.e., "can't intubate, can't ventilate").

The delivery of oxygen to the lungs through an over-the-needle catheter inserted through the skin into the trachea using a high pressure gas source is considered a form of conventional ventilation called percutaneous transtracheal ventilation (PTV).

Needle cricothyroidotomy differs from surgical cricothyroidotomy in that surgical cricothyroidotomy involves making an incision in the cricothyroid membrane and passing a tracheostomy or endotracheal tube through it into the trachea.

Needle cricothyroidotomy may be performed on patients of any age but is considered to be preferable to surgical cricothyroidotomy in infants and children up to 10 to 12 years of age because it is anatomically easier to perform with less potential damage to the larynx and surrounding structures.

However, surgical cricothyroidotomy provides more effective ventilation than needle cricothyroidotomy because of the larger diameter tube used and is typically chosen instead of needle cricothyroidotomy in adults and children over 10 to 12 years of age.

Indications for Use

The primary indication is inability to maintain the airway with noninvasive standard airway procedures (e.g., bag-valve-mask ventilation, endotracheal intubation) or rescue procedures (e.g., laryngeal mask airway).

Consider cricothyroidotomy to establish an airway in casualties having a total upper airway obstruction or inhalation burns preventing intubation or placement of a Combitube™.

Needle cricothyroidotomy with percutaneous transtracheal ventilation (PTV) should **NEVER** be used when the airway is maintainable through noninvasive means!

Gather pre-assembled cricothyroidotomy kit (every medic should have an easily accessible Cric Kit that contains all required items) or minimum essential equipment as below:

- Cutting instrument: #10 or 11 scalpel, knife blade
- 12-14 Gauge catheter-over-needle (e.g., Angiocath) with 10cc syringe attached for needle cricothyroidotomy (below). Syringe can also be used to inflate cuff on ET tube
- IV catheter 12-14 gauge (from above)
- ET tube
- cannula, or any non-collapsible tube that will allow sufficient airflow to maintain O2 saturation.

In a field setting, an ET tube is preferred because it is easy to secure. Use a size 6 -7 and insure that the cuff will hold air.

Other instruments:
- 2 Hemostats, needle holder
- tissue forceps
- scissors.
- Other supplies:
- Oxygen source and tubing
- BVM
- suctioning apparatus
- povidone-iodine prep
- gauze (preferably sterile)
- gloves(preferably sterile)
- blanket
- silk free ties (for bleeders; size 3-0)
- 3-0 silk suture material on a cutting needle

- Tape

Needle and Surgical Cricothyroidotomy

1. Place the casualty in the supine position (laying on their back) and place a rolled up blanket, poncho, shirts, or jackets under the casualty's neck or between the shoulder blades to hyperextend the casualty's neck and straighten the airway. ***WARNING: Do not hyperextend the casualty's neck if a cervical (neck) injury is suspected.***

2. Assemble needle/syringe set if not already done then locate and prep the cricothyroid membrane. Place a finger of your non-dominant hand on the thyroid cartilage (Adam's apple) and slide the finger down to find the cricoid cartilage.

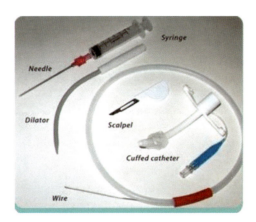

3. Palpate (feel) for the "V" notch of the thyroid cartilage. Slide the index finger down into the depression between the thyroid and cricoid cartilage, the cricothyroid membrane. Prep the skin over the membrane with povidone-iodine. Put on gloves (sterile if available) after assembling equipment and supplies.

Needle Cricothyroidotomy

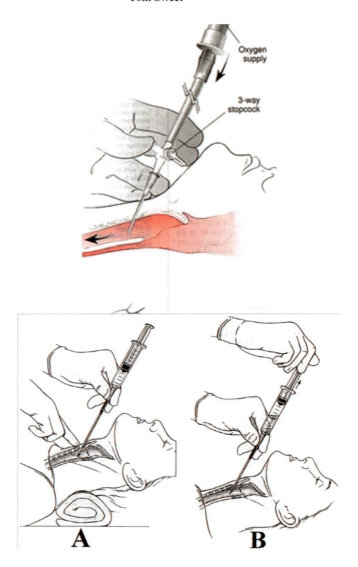

    a. Make a small nick in the skin with a #11 blade to open a hole for the IV catheter to slide through the skin

    b. Using the needle/catheter/syringe, penetrate the skin and fascia over the cricothyroid membrane at a $90°$ angle to the trachea while applying suction on the syringe. Advance the catheter through the cricothyroid membrane.

    c. Once air freely returns into the syringe, STOP advancement, and direct the needle toward the feet at a $45°$ angle.

    d. Hold the syringe in one hand, and use the other hand to advance the catheter off the needle towards the lower trachea.

e. Slide the catheter in up to the hub.

CAUTION: Do not release the catheter until it is adequately secured into place.

f. Check for air movement through the catheter by using the syringe to inject air through it and confirm free airflow. If air does not flow freely, straighten the tube and try again or withdraw the catheter and begin again at step b above.

g. If air flows freely and the patient is breathing on his own, use the 3-0 suture to make a stitch through the skin beside the catheter. Secure the catheter to the stitch with several knots. Connect catheter to an oxygen source at a flow rate of 50 psi or 15 L/min. See Steps below for wound care and on-going management.

h. If the patient is NOT breathing on his own, attach the syringe to the catheter, remove the plunger and deliver artificial respirations through the syringe and catheter. If the patient does not recover spontaneous respirations after several minutes, or if oxygen source is not available, proceed to **Surgical Cricothyroidotomy** below.

Surgical Cricothyroidotomy (If Needle cricothyroidotomy is not possible or is insufficient)

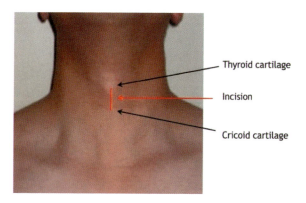

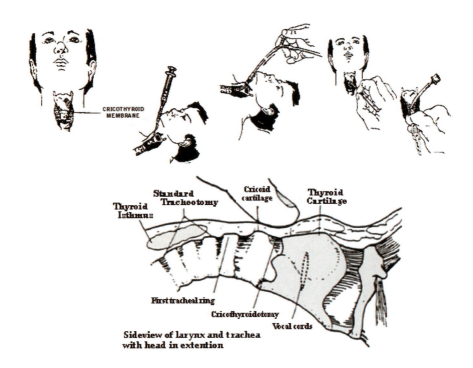

a. Proceed through the first three steps of **Needle Cricothyroidotomy** if not already done. Test ET cuff to ensure it holds air.

b. Raise the skin to form a tent-like appearance over the cricothyroid space, using the index finger and thumb.

c. With a cutting instrument in the dominant hand, make a 1 inch horizontal incision through the raised skin to the cricothyroid space.

CAUTION: Do not cut the cricothyroid membrane with this incision.

d. Relocate the cricothyroid space by touch and sight.

e. Stabilize the larynx with one hand and cut or poke a 1 inch incision through the cricothyroid membrane with the scalpel blade.

NOTE: A rush of air may be felt through the opening. Look for bilateral rise and fall of the chest.

f. Insert the ET tube or other airway tube through the opening into the trachea at a 90° angle to the trachea. Once in the trachea, direct the tube toward the feet at a 45° angle.

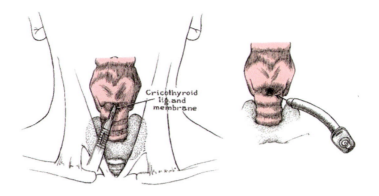

DO NOT insert an ET tube, or other long airway more than 3-4 inches to avoid intubating a single bronchus. Inflate the ET cuff if applicable.

DO NOT release the airway tube until it is secured (see below).

g. Connect the BVM to the tube and inflate the lungs, or have someone perform mouth to tube respirations. Auscultate the abdomen and both lung fields while observing for bilateral rise and fall of the chest. If there are bilateral breath sounds and bilateral rise and fall of the chest, the tube is properly placed and may be secured (see below). If not, reposition the tube as follows until adequate placement is obtained: (1) Unilateral breath sounds and unilateral rise or fall of the chest indicate that the tube is past the carina. Deflate the cuff on an ET tube, retract the tube 1-2 inches, inflate the ET cuff and recheck air exchange and placement. (2) Air coming out of the casualty's mouth indicates that the tube is pointed away from the lungs. Deflate the cuff on an ET tube, remove the tube, reinsert, inflate the cuff and recheck for air exchange and placement. (3) Any other problem indicates tube is not in the trachea. Follow the preceding step.

h. If air flows freely, and the patient is breathing on his own, proceed to next step. If the patient is **NOT** breathing on his own, continue providing respirations via the BVM with oxygen if available, or via mouth to tube assistance at the rate of about 20 breaths/min.

i. Secure the airway tube using tape (temporary), or use the 3-0 suture to make a stitch through the skin beside the tube. Secure the tube to the stitch with several knots.

j. Suction the casualty's airway, as necessary. Insert the suction catheter 4 to 5 inches into the tube. Apply suction only while withdrawing the catheter. Administer 1 cc of saline solution into the airway to loosen secretions and help facilitate suctioning.

NOTE: Ventilate the casualty several times or allow him to take several breaths between suctioning's.

Apply a dressing to further protect the tube or catheter and incision using one of the techniques below.

a. Cut two 4 X 4s or 4 X 8s halfway through. Place them on opposite sides of the tube so that the tube comes up through the cut and the gauze overlaps. Tape securely.

b. Apply a sterile dressing under the casualty's tube by making a V-shaped fold in a 4 X 8 gauze pad and placing it under the edge of the catheter to prevent irritation to the casualty. Tape securely.

Monitor casualty's respirations on a regular basis.

a. Reassess air exchange and placement every time the casualty is moved.

b. Assist respirations if respiratory rate falls below 12 or rises above 20 per minute.

What Not To Do:

DO NOT remove needle before advancing the catheter into trachea. (NEEDLE Cricothyroidotomy).

DO NOT forget to insure that the tube is correctly placed, and secured. (SURGICAL Cricothyroidotomy).

DO NOT fail to monitor your patient.

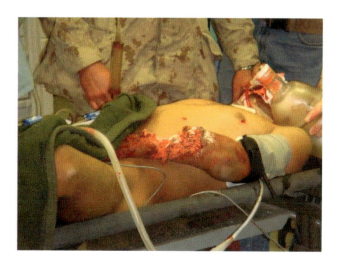

This is a 19-year-old Afghan truck driver who sustained extensive facial injuries and lost parts of his left forearm and left lower leg after a blast from an IED hit our convoy, causing extensive soft tissue, neurovascular and bone injury, and throwing him from the vehicle. I performed a surgical cricothyrotomy to secure the man's airway on the side of the road after pulling him from the line of fire during the attack.

4 PENETRATING CHEST TRAUMA

Penetrating chest trauma frequently creates serious or fatal injury because of the vital structures and processes that are housed within the chest cavity. Maintaining adequate pressures within the chest cavity is essential for adequate breathing.

The lungs are surrounded by thin, durable membranes called pleura. The parietal pleura lines the chest wall. The visceral pleura is attached to the surface of the lung. Between the two pleural layers is a small amount of fluid, which serves both as a lubricant and a means to provide surface tension to keep the lungs inflated. A fluid bond between the visceral and parietal pleura creates a steady pull between the two pleural layers, which leads to a constant intrapleural negative pressure.

The fluid bond is analogous to a water glass being placed upside down on a wet countertop. When the glass is pulled straight upward, the fluid bond creates a suction (negative pressure) and the glass can't be pulled upward off the countertop unless the fluid bond seal is broken.

The lung is comprised of fibers that have a natural recoil tendency. This recoil property wants to pull the lung inward away from the chest wall; however, the fluid bond in the pleural space overcomes this recoil and keeps the lungs from completely collapsing.

If the fluid bond were eliminated, the lungs would collapse to approximately 5% of their normal resting size. The integrity of the pleural layers and appropriate pressure within the chest are essential for adequate breathing. A break in the continuity and integrity of the pleural layer would reduce the fluid bond and allow the elastin recoil to collapse the lung.

It is believed that the pleural space can hold between 3–4 liters of blood or air. Air will cause a dramatic reduction in surface tension when the pleura lose contact with each other, resulting in the inability to expand the affected lung. The volume of blood that can collect in the pleural space is enough to cause exsanguination. Blood or other fluids in the pleural space can also cause alveolar collapse in the areas where these substances are present.

It should be noted that during deep exhalation, the diaphragm rises as high as T4/T5. This means that an injury in the area of diaphragmatic movement may involve the chest, abdomen or both.

A final issue with anatomy is that many fail to consider the patient's "upper back" part of the chest cavity. The upper back is actually the posterior of the chest cavity and must be considered during assessment and care of the patient, especially in the event of penetrating trauma leading to pneumothorax or tension pneumothorax.

Pneumothorax (Sucking Chest Wound)

A pneumothorax occurs when the integrity of the chest wall is compromised allowing air to enter, frequently caused by a penetrating wound. However, a pneumothorax may also occur spontaneously or due to a medical condition. In this case, we are limiting discussion to the penetrating chest injury.

When an opening is created between the outside environment and the pleural space, intrathoracic and environmental pressures have a tendency to attempt to equalize. With the break in the pleural fluid bond (discussed earlier), the ability of the injured pleura and lung to expand is severely limited.

The extent of the pneumothorax can vary greatly, depending on the type of wound, location of the wound and whether the wound seals itself spontaneously.

Be sure to auscultate (listen to) the chest thoroughly. Percussion over the hyper inflated pleura will produce a tympanic or hollow sound known as hyper resonance. A decrease in breath sounds and hyper resonance may be heard only over the apices in small pneumothoraces; thus, be sure to assess this area thoroughly.

A significant complication of a pneumothorax is development of a tension pneumothorax.

This occurs when a pneumothorax causes air to build up in the pleural space on the injured side, leading to a significant increase in pressure on one side of the chest. This can occur when an open pneumothorax seals itself and air continues to escape from the injured lung, or when tissue associated with an open chest wound creates a flutter valve effect, allowing air to enter but sealing the wound when air attempts to escape. The lung on the affected side will usually collapse.

As pressure builds on the injured side of the chest, it begins to cause a shift of the mediastinum toward the uninjured side of the chest. This shift begins to compress the uninjured lung and also may kink the inferior and superior venae cava, reducing venous return to the right side of the heart.

The reduction in venous return will reduce the preload of the left ventricle, leading to a decrease in cardiac output and consequential poor perfusion and hypotension. Thus, a tension pneumothorax creates not only a respiratory compromise but also a cardiovascular compromise.

Tension pneumothorax presents with respiratory distress, jugular venous distention (JVD), diminished breath sounds, tachycardia and narrow pulse pressure.

Although tracheal deviation and jugular venous distention are commonly cited signs of this condition, they both occur late in the condition. It is difficult to detect tracheal deviation at a level above the suprasternal notch; however, it is usually easier to palpate a shift in the trachea than to see it.

The illustration below list the most common signs and symptoms of a Tension Pneumothorax.

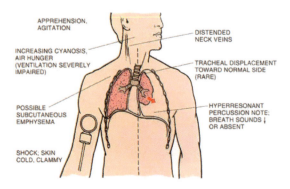

Hemothorax

A hemothorax is a collection of blood in the pleural space. As noted above, this space will hold between 3–4 liters of blood. Although blood in this capacity will prevent gas exchange due to alveolar collapse, it also can cause death from blood loss without one drop of blood ever leaving the body. This means that hemothorax can affect the body in two ways: bleeding and by impeding gas exchange in the lungs.

The blood from hemothorax can come from two general areas: extrapleural and intrapleural, which includes the great vessels of the body in the mediastinum. The most common and often most profuse bleeding is caused by laceration of the extrapleural intercostal or internal mammary arteries.

On the underside of each rib, and slightly toward the inside, is a vein, artery and nerve. This is important to remember in regards to placement of decompression needles.

Intrapleurally, bleeding from damage to the lung parenchyma is usually limited because of self-compression and the relative low pressures in these vessels. Of course, a rupture of the great vessels contained in the mediastinum, including the aorta and the superior and inferior venae cava, will cause a massive hemothorax.

When assessing the patient with a hemothorax, you will likely find signs of hypovolemic shock and a mechanism of injury consistent with penetrating chest injury to include GSW, stabbing or even a closed chest injury, if it causes injuries to blood vessels.

In hemothorax, you would find a dull sound on percussion over affected areas. It is important to note that many of these patients are placed laying down, which may diminish the accuracy of auscultation or percussion, especially in minor to moderate hemothorax, by causing a distribution of the blood over a greater area, masking pertinent physical findings.

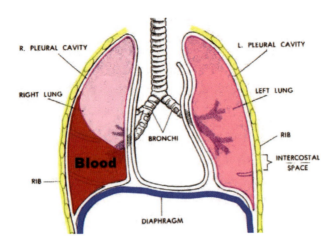

Needle Decompression

A needle thoracostomy can be performed faster than a tube thoracostomy in a rapidly deteriorating patient having signs of a tension pneumothorax. This can be life-saving and gives enough relief to provide time for you to insert a chest tube. Once the chest tube is properly inserted, remove the needle.

You will need to have the following supplies ready before you perform the needle decompression or chest tube placement:

- 18 gauge needle
- 16-18 gauge IV Catheter
- 10-20 cc syringe
- sterile saline
- alcohol pads,
- Betadine
- latex gloves (sterile if possible)
- assorted chest tubes (sizes 28-32 French for adult, 36-40 French for adult with hemothorax, 12-14 French for children)
- water seal drainage system (e.g., Pleur-Evac) and
- connection tubing for suction (alternate: one-way valve made from finger of latex glove)

Instruments:
- scalpel

- forceps
- gauze (may be in prepared tray)
- Lidocaine 1-2 % without epinephrine (if available; **DO NOT** delay decompression or chest tube insertion for anesthesia if patient is in severe distress or unconscious)
- petrolatum gauze
- external dressing (4x4)
- adhesive tape

You can find Chest Decompression "kits", like the ones in the picture below and the next page, at www.vanguardsurvival.com and other merchants both on and off line.

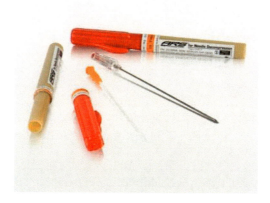

The ThoraQuick Needle Decompression kit is in use with British Special Operations and is one of the best solutions for chest decompression in the conditions you will likely find in a survival/SHTF situation.

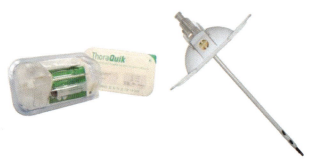

Before you do anything else Figure out which lung has the pneumothorax! Insure that the procedure is performed on the side suspected of having a pneumothorax (tension pneumothorax, simple pneumothorax, hemothorax), which will be the lung without breath sounds. Hyper-resonance is also a helpful sign, but the lack of breath sounds after penetrating or blunt trauma is a definitive sign.

Needle Thoracostomy (Needle Decompression)

1. Prep the chest wall by pouring Betadine over the intended site or swab with an alcohol wipe.

2. Insert an 18 Ga (or larger) 1.5 inch needle or IV catheter into the 2nd intercostal space, along the mid-clavicular line (an imaginary line from the middle of the collarbone, or clavicle; the interspace immediately below the clavicle is the 1st interspace). Run your finger down the mid-clavicular line, over the 2nd rib, to the 2nd intercostal space. Insert the IV catheter immediately above the 3rd rib.

3. This will release a rush of air from the pressure built up in the pleural space. Advance the catheter up to the hub, then remove the needle stylet and discard. The patient's ability to spontaneously breathe usually improves immediately. Leave the catheter in place, and attach a three-way stopcock, which can be used to drain air as it accumulates

4. This can improve the patient's symptoms and be life-saving. Primarily, it is fast and easy to perform, providing enough time for you to set up for inserting a chest tube. The life-threatening emergency is the tension pneumothorax, not the simple pneumothorax that remains.

5. Once the chest tube is properly inserted, the catheter can be removed.

Alternative Technique

Remove the plunger from a 10-20 cc syringe filled with sterile saline, attach an 18 gauge needle/catheter (or larger) and use it to perform the thoracostomy. This allows handling of the needle/IV catheter more precisely and provides visual "bubbles" when the trapped air is released into the syringe. This is helpful in a noisy environment.

Once the catheter is placed and the needle removed, setup for chest tube can begin. If the location is not safe for the second procedure, leave the catheter in place, attach a three-way stopcock to drain air as it accumulates, cover the catheter with gauze and tape, and move to a secure location for the procedure.

Tube Thoracostomy (Chest Tube)

Tube thoracostomy is the insertion of a tube (chest tube) into the pleural cavity to drain air, blood, bile, pus, or other fluids. Whether the accumulation of air or fluid is the result of rapid traumatic filling with air or blood placement of a chest tube allows for continuous, large volume drainage until the underlying pathology can be more formally addressed. The list of specific treatable etiologies is extensive (see Indications), but without intervention, patients are at great risk for major morbidity or mortality.

Indications

- Pneumothorax -Open or closed
- Simple or tension
- Hemothorax
- Hemopneumothorax
- Patients with penetrating chest wall injury who are intubated or about to be intubated

There are many other indications for chest tube placement that we will not cover because they are not relevant to the purposes of this book.

Equipment

- Chest tube drainage device with water
- Suction source (optional) and tubing
- Sterile gloves
- Betadine solution
- Sterile drapes
- Surgical marker
- Lidocaine 1% with epinephrine
- Syringes, 10-20 mL (2)
- Needle, 25 gauge (ga), 5/8 in
- Needle, 23 ga, 1.5 in; or 27 ga, 1.5 in; for instilling local anesthesia
- Blade, No. 10, on a handle
- Large and medium Kelly clamps
- Large curved Mayo scissors
- Large straight suture scissors
- Silk or nylon suture, 0 or 1-0
- Needle driver
- Vaseline gauze
- Gauze squares, 4 x 4 in (10)
- Sterile adhesive tape, 4 in wide
- Chest tube of appropriate size
  - Man - 28-32F
  - Woman - 28F
  - Child - 12-28F
  - Infant - 12-16F
  - Neonate - 10-12F

Water Seal Drainage Systems

The chest tube is connected to a glass tube placed in a bottle containing water. The glass tube extends below the water level, therefore, the name sealed drainage. The water seal prevents air from getting back into the chest. As the patient inhales, the chest cavity expands, pushing air and drainage from the chest, into the tubes, and ultimately into the bottle.

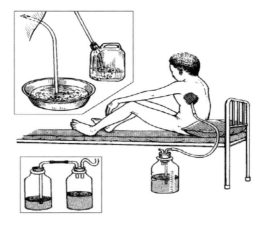

The chest tube is connected to a glass tube submerged 2cm below the water level in a capped, covered bottle. The rubber cap fits tightly around the two glass tubes to prevent air from getting into the system. There is always an air vent in the top of the bottle to allow air to escape. Never cover the air vent in any system.

A one bottle uses gravity only. It is never hooked up to a suction machine. Inspiration forces air through the chest tube, so therefore, a few bubbles are seen coming up through the water.

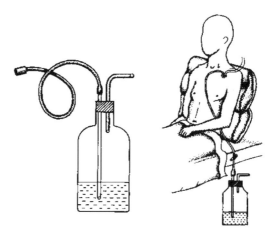

The water in the glass tube oscillates during the respiratory cycle. It should rise on   inspiration and fall on expiration (up on in, down on out). All chest bottle systems must be will secured so that they are not knocked over and must always remain below the level of the client's chest.

This system is used primarily with pneumothorax where a lot of drainage is not expected. If the bottle fills up with drainage, it will require more effort for the client to expel air and fluid from the pleural cavity.

To demonstrate this, take a straw and put it in the bottom of a full glass of liquid. Now blow bubbles through the straw. Take and move the straw to one inch below the surface liquid, now blow bubbles. More effort is needed to blow bubbles when the straw is at the bottom of the glass.

Chest Tube Insertion

Patient Position

The preferred position for drain insertion is on the bed, slightly rotated, with the arm on the effected side behind the patient's head to expose the axillary area. An alternative is for the patient to sit upright leaning over an adjacent table with a pillow or bent at the waist as far as possible. Insertion should be in the "safe triangle" illustrated below.

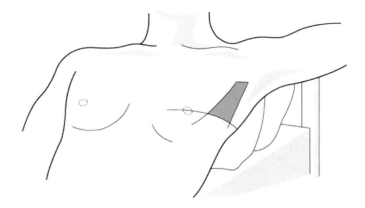

Drain Insertion Site

The most common position for chest tube insertion is in the mid axillary line through the "safe triangle" illustrated and described above. This position minimizes risk to underlying structures such as the internal mammary artery and avoids damage to muscle and breast tissue resulting in unsightly scarring. Generally, the tube is placed in the 3rd to 5th intercostal space on the mid-axillary line. As illustrated on the next page.

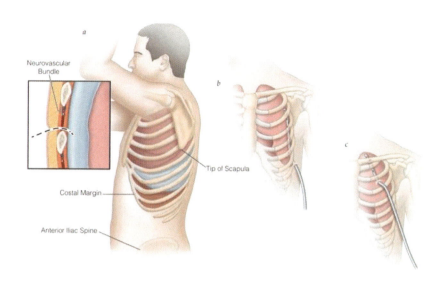

Placing the Chest Tube

Position the patient as described above. Identify the fifth intercostal and the midaxillary line.

- The skin incision is made in between the midaxillary and anterior axillary lines over a rib that is below the intercostal level selected for chest tube insertion.
- A surgical marker can be used to better delineate the anatomy.

Prep the chest wall by pouring Betadine over the intended site. Site of insertion: along the mid-axillary line (a line running straight down from the middle of the armpit), always above the level of nipples in males (5th intercostal space since below this level there is a risk of puncturing the diaphragm). For a better idea of where you are going to make the incision refer to the picture below.

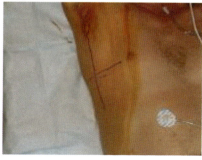

Infiltrate 1% lidocaine along the track to be used. Generally, the tube is placed in the 3rd to 5th intercostal space on the mid-axillary line. Use the 25-ga needle to inject 5 mL of the local anesthetic solution into the skin overlying the initial skin incision, as shown below.

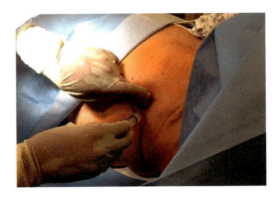

Use the longer needle (23 or, preferably, 27 ga) to infiltrate about 5 mL of the anesthetic solution to a wide area of subcutaneous tissue superior to the expected initial incision. Redirect the needle to the expected course of the chest tube (following the upper border of the rib below the fifth intercostal space), and inject approximately 10 mL of the anesthetic solution into the periosteum (if bone is encountered), intercostal muscle, and the pleura.

Aspiration of air, blood, pus, or a combination thereof into the syringe confirms that the needle entered the pleural cavity.

Use the No. 11 or 10 blade to make a skin incision approximately 3-4 cm long over the rib that is below the desired intercostal level of entry. ***DO NOT*** cut into the intercostal space itself! The skin incision should be in the same direction as the rib itself.

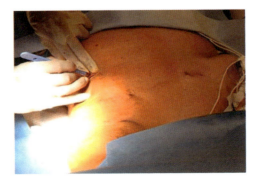

Insert a large curved hemostat (Kelly Clamp) with the curve pointed toward the ribs and create a tunnel over the top of the rib. This tunnel helps to stabilize and seal the chest tube after placement. Curve the clamp over the top of the rib. Advance it slowly, opening and closing the jaws of the hemostat to clear a path and then puncture into the thoracic cavity. **_DO NOT_** advance straight in.

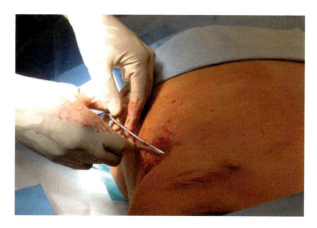

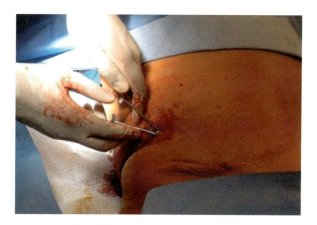

Palpate the tract with a finger as shown in the picture on the next page, and make sure that the tract ends at the upper border of the rib above the skin incision. Insertion of the chest tube as close as possible to the upper border of the rib will minimize the risks of injury to the nerve and blood vessels that follow the lower border of each rib.

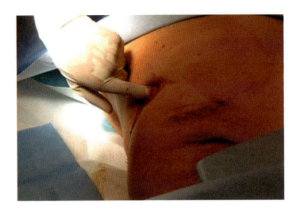

Adding more local anesthetic to the intercostal muscles and pleura at this time is recommended.

Use a closed large Kelly clamp to pass through the intercostal muscles and parietal pleura and enter into the pleural space, as shown below.

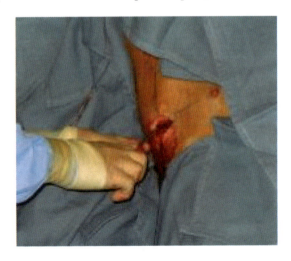

This maneuver requires some force and twisting motion of the tip of the closed Kelly clamp.

This motion should be done in a controlled manner so the instrument does not enter too far into the chest, which could injure the lung or diaphragm.

Upon entry into the pleural space, a rush of air or fluid should occur.

- The Kelly clamp should be opened (while still inside the pleural space) and then withdrawn so that its jaws enlarge the dissected tract through all layers of the chest wall as shown. This facilitates passage of the chest tube when it is inserted.

Use a sterile, gloved finger to appreciate the size of the tract and to feel for lung tissue and possible adhesions, as shown in the image below. Rotate the finger 360° to appreciate the presence of dense adhesions that cannot be broken and require placement of the chest tube in a different site.

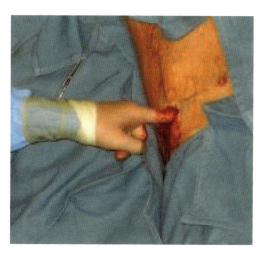

Measure the length between the skin incision and the apex of the lung to estimate how far the chest tube should be inserted.

If desired, place a clamp over the tube to mark the estimated length.

Grasp the proximal (fenestrated) end of the chest tube with the large Kelly clamp and introduce it through the tract and into the thoracic cavity as shown.

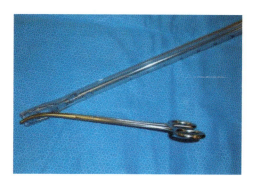

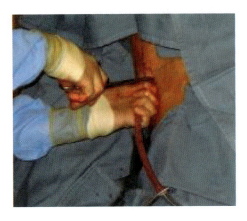

Release the Kelly clamp and continue to advance the chest tube posteriorly and superiorly. Make sure that all of the fenestrated holes in the chest tube are inside the thoracic cavity.

Connect the chest tube to the drainage device as shown (some prefer to cut the distal end of the chest tube to facilitate its connection to the drainage device tubing). Release the cross clamp that is on the chest tube only after the chest tube is connected to the drainage device.

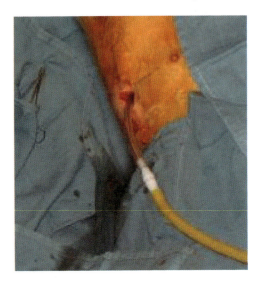

Before securing the tube with stitches, look for a respiration-related swing in the fluid level of the water seal device, described above, to confirm correct intrathoracic placement.

In emergency conditions, use a one-way Heimlich valve instead. Cut a finger off of a latex glove. Fasten it as air-tightly as possible over the end of the tube: insert the free end of the chest tube inside the open end of the glove finger and tape the glove finger around the tube. Cut a 2 cm slit in the closed end of the glove finger. Or use a 5"-6" length of Penrose tubing that is secured as airtight as possible to the end of the tube.

This will allow air to escape, but the glove finger will collapse on inspiration and prevent air from entering the lung. This will also collect blood draining from the chest tube.

Secure the chest tube to the skin using 0 or 1-0 silk or nylon stitches, as depicted below.

Diagram illustrating 'purse string' closure stitch

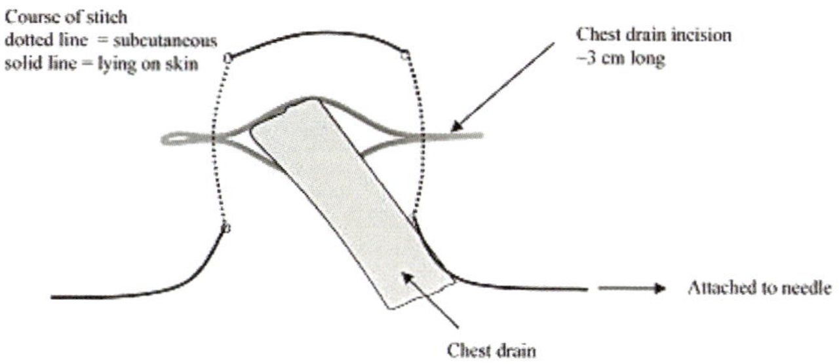

Course of stitch
dotted line = subcutaneous
solid line = lying on skin

Chest drain incision ~3 cm long

Attached to needle

Chest drain

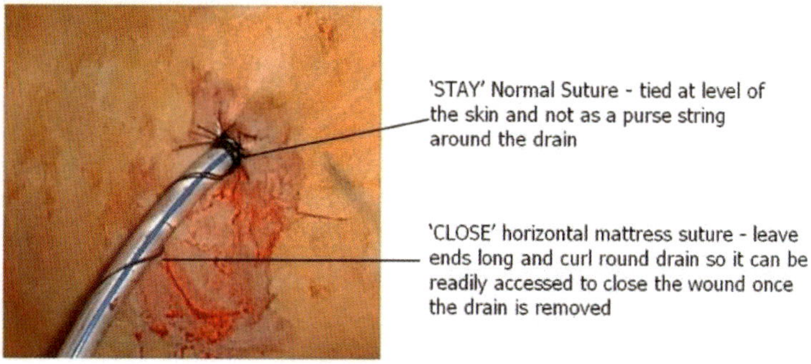

'STAY' Normal Suture - tied at level of the skin and not as a purse string around the drain

'CLOSE' horizontal mattress suture - leave ends long and curl round drain so it can be readily accessed to close the wound once the drain is removed

Securing sutures: Two separate through-and-through, simple, interrupted stitches on each side of the chest tube are recommended. This technique ensures tight closure of the skin incision and prevents routine patient movements from dislodging the chest tube.

Each stitch should be tightly tied to the skin, then wrapped tightly around the chest tube several times to cause slight indentation, and then tied again.

Sealing suture: A central vertical mattress stitch with ends left long and knotted together can be placed to allow for sealing of the tract once the chest tube is removed.

Place Vaseline-impregnated gauze around the tube at the incision site, cover over that with 4x4 gauze and tape in place. The Vaseline gauze will prevent air leaks.

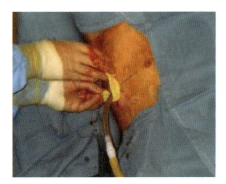

Create an occlusive dressing to place over the chest tube by turning regular gauze squares (4 x 4 in) into Y-shaped fenestrated gauze squares and using 4-in adhesive tape to secure them to the chest wall, as shown below. Make sure to provide enough padding between the chest tube and the chest wall.

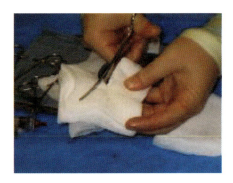

Strap the emerging chest tube on to the lower trunk with a "mesentery" fold of adhesive tape, as this avoids kinking of the tube as it passes through the chest wall. It also helps reduce wound site pain and discomfort for the patient. All connections are then taped in their long axis to avoid disconnections.

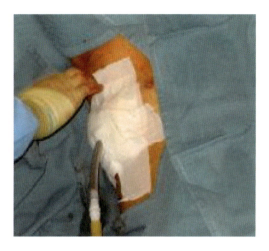

The picture below shows a chest tube I initially placed in the field following an ambush of our convoy by Taliban insurgents on the highway between Kandahar and Kabul in 2007. The bullet struck him in the back just below the shoulder blade and did not exit as he was attempting to drive out of the Kill Zone.

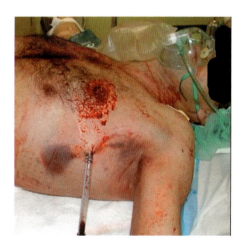

Things to Keep in Mind

In cases of high-pressure empyema or pleural effusion, removal of 50-200 mL of fluid using a syringe and a 14-ga needle, as shown below, might prevent high-pressure spraying of the accumulated fluid once the pleural space is entered with the surgical instrument.

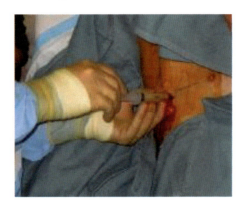

Since the intercostal vessels and nerve run on the bottom side of each rib, incision and tunneling should be performed over the rib. Insertion of the chest tube should be performed immediately above and as close to the superior rib margin as possible in order to minimize the risks of injury to the nerve and blood vessels that follow the lower margin of each rib.

Errors that are commonly observed but easily avoidable include inadequate volume of local anesthetic, failure to wait adequate time for anesthetic to take effect, and too small an incision.

Small-bore drains are recommended, as they are more comfortable than larger-bore tubes, but no evidence indicates that one is superior to the other. Large-bore drains are recommended for drainage of acute hemothorax and to monitor further blood loss.

Complications Associated with Chest Tube Placement

Minor complications of chest tube placement such as unresolved/re-accumulation of pneumothorax or misplacement of the tube (too deep/kinked) are common and approach approximately 30% according to the American College of Trauma Surgeons.

Improper placement

Horizontal (over the diaphragm) - Acceptable for hemothorax; should be repositioned for pneumothorax.

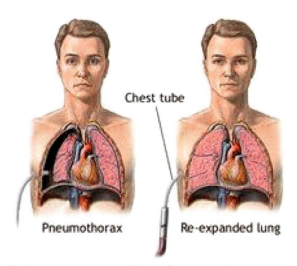

If the patient's condition does not improve, or deteriorates, the placement of the tube is suspect and it should be checked thoroughly for proper placement, or repositioned.

If there is a persistent pneumothorax despite a properly placed chest tube, consider increasing the column of water by 5 cm increments up to 30 cm before inserting a second chest tube.

Prior to removal, the chest tube should be clamped for 2-4 hours or longer. If there is no re-accumulation of air, the chest tube can be removed.

What Not To Do

Do not insert a chest tube if a tension pneumothorax is suspected and the patient is rapidly deteriorating— perform a needle thoracostomy instead for rapid relief.

Do not reposition or remove and replace a suspect tube if the patient shows signs of a repeat tension pneumothorax. Perform a second needle thoracentesis, then insert a second chest tube.

Considerations for Chest Tube Placement in Children

In general, treat a small (< 25%), simple pneumothorax conservatively, unless the patient is significantly symptomatic. Consider using 100% oxygen via a non-rebreathing face mask (if available) to increase reabsorption of intrapleural air; however, the potential for oxygen toxicity should be considered, and this treatment should not be continued for long periods.

The patient should be observed to look for improvement.

A small, simple pneumothorax in a patient who experienced trauma is best treated with a chest tube, because the condition may rapidly convert into a tension pneumothorax, especially if positive pressure ventilation is applied.

Large or significantly symptomatic pneumothoraces require chest tube placement and surgical intervention. A tension pneumothorax requires immediate decompression with needle thoracostomy.

In addition, the chest tube wound site should be monitored for infection and to ensure proper healing.

Complications

Complications directly related to pneumothorax are few. Recognition and proper treatment of a pneumothorax are needed to prevent expansion, hypoxia (with its complications), and tension with subsequent cardiovascular collapse and death.

Chest tube insertion may result in significant bleeding, infection, or both. Insertion too far below the recommended fourth or fifth intercostal space may result in intra-abdominal placement, with possible abdominal visceral or diaphragmatic injury.

The illustration on the following page shows the proper technique for placing a chest tube in a pediatric patient.

Landmarks for chest tube insertion.

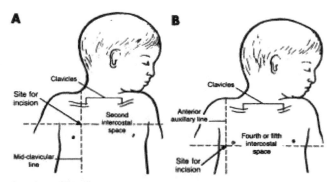

Insertion of Chest Tube

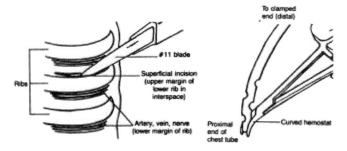

Securing the Chest Tube

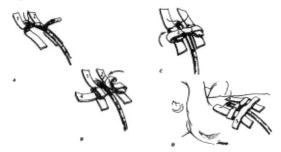

Pericardiocentesis

The patient has sustained a penetrating wound in the chest that may have entered the heart covering (pericardium), and is showing signs of shock – hypotension (low blood pressure), tachycardia (rapid heart rate), and tachypnea (rapid breathing) with narrowed pulse pressure, muffled heart sounds, pulses paradoxicus (heart rate increasing with expiration, decreasing with inspiration–greater than normally seen).

You must be aware that this procedure is dangerous and should not be attempted without prior training, and only as a last resort in life threatening emergencies when vital signs deteriorate: (narrow pulse pressure) low mean arterial pressure, +/- muffled heart sounds.

If the vital signs are stable, you should continue IV fluids 9which we will cover in the next chapter) and monitor the patient only. There are also more rare etiologies for developing fluid (viral pericarditis), as well as air (pneumopericardium in diving) in the pericardial sac. These conditions can be relieved with the same procedure outlined below to relieve blood in the pericardial sac.

You will need

- 18 gauge spinal needle or Pericardiocentesis kit with Mansfield catheter
- 60cc syringe
- Sterile preparation kit (alcohol wipe may be adequate in emergencies)
- Local anesthetic (Lidocaine w/ or w/o Epinephrine)
- Sterile needles
- 3-way stopcock
- Gauze pads/bandage
- Emergency drugs (atropine, lidocaine, epinephrine, oxygen)

Position the patient in a semi-recumbent position at a 30- to 45-degree angle. This position brings the heart closer to the anterior chest wall. The supine position is an acceptable alternative.

There are two options for Pericardiocentesis under the **EXTREME EMERGENCY conditions once TSHTF.**

Option A - Emergency Technique to Withdraw Fluid Once

1. Clean sub-xiphoid area with antiseptic solution (Betadine)
2. Connect 18 gauge spinal needle and 60 cc syringe
3. Place your finger 0.5 cm below the costal margin of the patient's xiphoid to mark the point of needle insertion.
4. Raise the needle to a 30° angle from parallel to the patient's chest. Aim the needle at the tip of the ipsilateral (same side) scapula (shoulder blade)
5. Insert the needle, maintaining slight suction and advanced until blood flow is obtained, and then stop advancement.
6. Withdraw as much a blood as possible and then withdraw the needle. Only a small amount (5-10 cc) removed can have a marked improvement in vital signs.

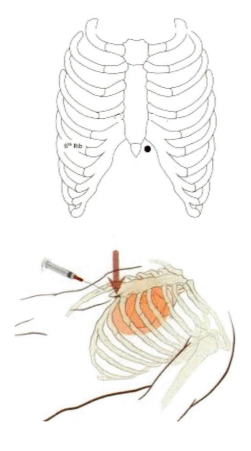

Option B - Technique to Withdraw Fluid Multiple Times

1. Attach a central line needle and catheter to a 60 cc syringe.
2. Follow the procedure as above.
3. When fluid is obtained, hold the syringe and needle in one hand, and gently advance (slide) the catheter into the pericardial space.
4. Withdraw the needle from the catheter.
5. Attach the 3-way stopcock (closed position) to the hub of the catheter.
6. Remove the needle from the syringe and discard. Connect one end of IV tubing to one port of the 3 way stopcock, the other end of the IV tubing attach to a 60 cc syringe (optional to connect another IV line to the third port of the stopcock for ejecting blood from the syringe).
7. Open the 3 way stopcock to the syringe to withdraw fluid from the pericardial space, then turn open to ejection port IV line to eject the fluid out.
8. When no further fluid/blood return, turn the 3-way stopcock to closed or in-between position

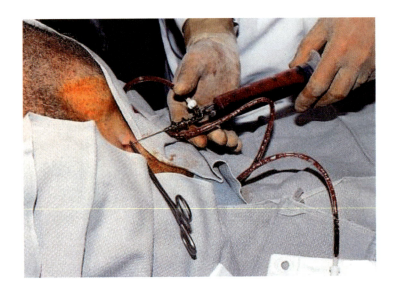

Care must be taken not to insert the needle more than 1/16th -1/8th of an inch once blood is obtained.

The catheter can be left in if the medic has a catheter line that can be switched between closed and open.

Remember, small movements of the syringe can have large effects on movement of the tip of the needle causing lacerations of the myocardium or coronary arteries.

Pericardiocentesis should only be used in an extreme emergency since even the slightest deviation or slip can cause more damage or death.

5 FLUID RESESITATION

The treatment of patients with hypovolemic (low blood volume) shock often begins at an accident scene or at home. You should work to prevent further injury, transport the patient to the hospital as rapidly as possible, and initiate appropriate treatment in the field.

Direct pressure should be applied to external bleeding vessels to prevent further blood loss.

Two large-bore IV lines should be started. The Poiseuille law states that flow is inversely related to the length of the IV catheter and directly related to its radius to the fourth power.

Thus, a short large-bore IV catheter is ideal; the bore is much more significant than the length. IV access may be obtained by means of percutaneous access in the antecubital veins, cutdown of saphenous or arm veins, which we will cover a little later in the chapter.

Intraosseous access has and continues to be used for hypotensive children younger than 6 years, though Intraosseous access has also been used to great effect on the battlefield in recent years. The most important factor in determining the route of access is your skill and experience.

Once IV access is obtained, initial fluid resuscitation is performed with an isotonic crystalloid, such as lactated Ringer solution or normal saline. An initial bolus of 1-2 L is given in an adult (20 mL/kg in a pediatric patient), and the patient's response is assessed.

If vital signs return to normal, the patient may be monitored to ensure stability, and blood should be sent for typed and cross-matched. If vital signs transiently improve, crystalloid infusion should continue and type-specific blood obtained. If little or no improvement is seen, crystalloid infusion should continue, and type O blood should be given (type O Rh-negative blood should be given to female patients of childbearing age to prevent sensitization and future complications).

If a patient is moribund and markedly hypotensive (class IV shock), both crystalloid and type O blood, if available, should be started initially. These guidelines for crystalloid and blood infusion are not rules; therapy should be based on the condition of the patient.

The position of the patient can be used to improve circulation; one example is raising the hypotensive patient's legs while fluid is being given. Another example of useful positioning is rolling a hypotensive pregnant patient with trauma onto her left side, which displaces the fetus from the inferior vena cava and increases circulation.

The Trendelenburg (head down, feet up) position is no longer recommended for hypotensive patients, as the patient is predisposed to aspiration. In addition, the Trendelenburg position does not improve cardiopulmonary performance and may worsen gas exchange.

Controlling further blood loss

Control of further hemorrhage depends on the source of bleeding and often requires surgical intervention. In the patient with trauma, external bleeding should be controlled with direct pressure, elevation, pressure dressings, and/or tourniquets'; internal bleeding requires surgical intervention. Long-bone fractures should be treated with traction to decrease blood loss.

Restoring normal circulating volume and BP prior to definitive control of bleeding

During World War I, Cannon observed and characterized patients in clinical shock. He later suggested a model of permissive hypotension in the treatment of torso wounds, with the intent of minimizing further bleeding.

Findings from early studies showed that animals that were bled had increased survival if they received fluid resuscitation. However, in these studies, bleeding was well controlled with ligation after the animals were bled.

During the Korean and Vietnam wars, much more aggressive fluid resuscitation, as well as rapid access to definitive care, was emphasized. It was noted that patients who were aggressively resuscitated tended to have better outcomes, and in the 1970s, these principles were widely adopted in civilian patients.

Since then, many studies have been conducted to determine if these principles are valid in patients with uncontrolled hemorrhage. Most of these studies revealed increased survival in the permissive hypotension or delayed treatment arms. The theory is that increased pressure causes more bleeding and disrupts initial clots, whereas extreme hypotension may increase the risk of cerebral perfusion.

The questions that have not been answered adequately are as follows: Which mechanisms and injury patterns are more amenable to the restoration of circulating blood volume? What BP is adequate but not excessive?

Although some data indicate that a systolic BP of 80-90 mm Hg may be adequate in penetrating truncal trauma without head injury, further studies are needed.

Current recommendations are for aggressive fluid resuscitation with lactated Ringer solution or normal saline in all patients with signs and symptoms of shock, regardless of underlying cause.

Starting an IV

All necessary equipment should be prepared, assembled and available prior to starting the IV.

Basic equipment includes:
- Gloves
- Appropriate size catheter 14-22 GA IV catheter
- Non-latex tourniquet
- Alcohol swab/other cleaning instrument
- 2x2 or 4x4 gauze
- 6x7cm Tegaderm™ Transparent Dressing (if available)
- 3-4 pieces of 2.5 cm tape approximately 10 cm in length
- IV bag with solution set (tubing) (flushed and ready) or saline lock

The pictures on the next page show the basic supplies need for an IV.

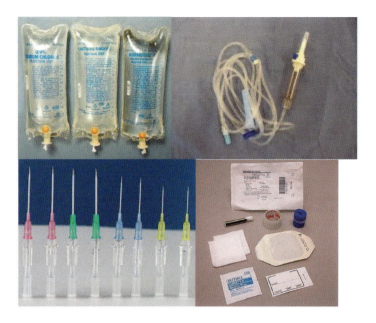

To prepare the IV line, protective caps are removed from the fluid bag and the spiked end of the IV tubing.

The regulating clamp for the IV line should be closed. The spiked end of the IV tubing is inserted into the receptacle on the IV bag while holding the IV bag inverted.

The bag is then held upright with the IV line hanging from the bottom. The drip chamber should be filled half-way by pinching it and releasing.

Following this the bag should be hung at a point above the patient, and the regulating clamp should be opened to "flush" the line of air bubbles prior to connection to the patient.

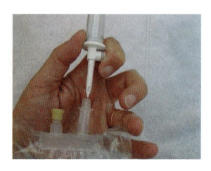

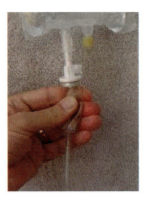

The first step in the process is to find a good vein to insert the IV. The large vein located in the bend of the elbow is most often used, but nurses can also find good vein sites on the forearm, feet, scalp, hand, and wrist if necessary.

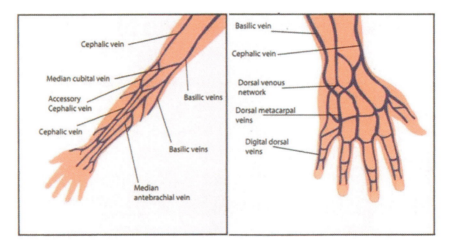

Apply a tourniquet high on the upper arm. It should be tight enough to visibly indent the skin without causing patient discomfort. In order to maximize venous engorgement, have the patient squeeze his hand into a fist several times.

Now start the search for suitable distended subcutaneous veins. If you cannot see any veins popping up from the distention caused by the tourniquet, you can sometimes feel them by palpating the arm. If you still cannot find any veins, then it might be useful to cover the arm in a warm compress to help with peripheral vasodilation.

If after a meticulous search no veins are found; release the tourniquet

Advanced First Aid for Survival

from above the elbow, place it around the forearm and search in the distal forearm, wrist and hand. If no suitable veins are found, then you will have to move to the other arm. Be careful to stay away from arteries which are pulsatile.

Once a suitable vein is found, then it is necessary to clean and disinfect the area by swiping it several times with two alcohol wipes. If the arm is particularly hairy in this spot it may be necessary to use a disposable razor to shave the hair partially too make a region that will be clean.

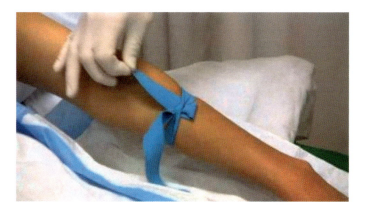

Usually a 14 or 16 gauge angiocatheter is suitable. Take it apart and put it back together to get a sense of how it works and how much force is required to slide the plastic catheter over the metal stylet.

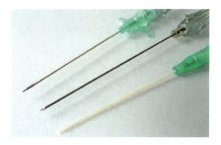

Use one hand to apply counter tension against the skin. This hand, generally the left hand, will be pulling the skin distally towards the wrist in the opposite direction to the needle will be advancing.

When applying counter tension be careful not to compress inflow to the vein which may cause the vein to collapse. With the bevel UP advance the angiocatheter through the skin over top of the vein or adjacent to the vein.

Use a quick, jab motion to minimize patient discomfort. Slow pokes through the skin will maximize the sensation of pain. Then advance the angiocatheter well into the vein and look for the dark red flashback of blood at the angio catheter hub indicating that the angio catheter is within the vein.

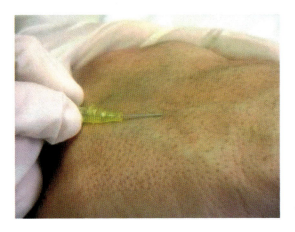

If this first pass is unsuccessful in entering the vein and there is no flashback then slowly withdraw the angio catheter, without pulling all the way out, and carefully watch for the flashback to occur. If you are still not within the vein, then advance it again in a 2nd attempt to enter the vein.

While withdrawing always stop before pulling all the way out to avoid repeating the painful initial skin puncture. If after several manipulations the vein is never entered and the attempt is considered a failure; release the tourniquet, place a gauze over the skin puncture site, withdraw the angiocatheter and tape down the gauze. Now it is time to move onto the other arm and try again.

Once the angiocatheter is well seated within the vein, slide the plastic angio catheter forward deeper into the vein over top of the needle. The hub of the angio catheter should be all the way to the skin puncture site. The plastic catheter should slide forward easily. Do not force!!

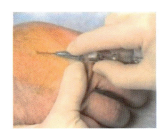

Attach the male end of the drip set to the female hub of the angio catheter. Lock the iv tubing to the angio catheter by advancing and rotating the luer-locking mechanism. It requires a clockwise twist to fully lock.

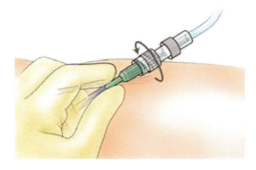

At this point, quickly test the IV by removing the tourniquet and opening the clamp to make sure it is working properly. The fluid should flush easily.

If the fluid does not flush easily, check to be sure the tourniquet is released. Also try straightening the arm because sometimes bending the elbow can kink a vein and prevent the iv from functioning.

If it still does not flush easily, try aspirating. Sometimes an iv will begin to work if it is withdrawn slightly so the tip of the iv seats in a better position within the vein.

Tape the IV in place using the Tegaderm or three or four strips of tape to prevent accidental removal. Place one or two pieces over the actual skin puncture site.

Place additional pieces over loops of tubing so that there is some strain relief. Consider taping to be one of the most important tasks because it prevents you from having to repeat the IV insertion in the event of an inadvertent tug on the IV tubing.

The pictures on the next page show different ways to secure an IV in place.

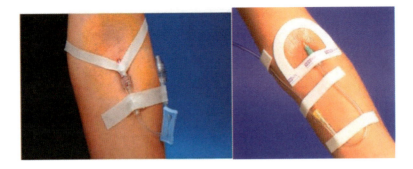

Once the IV is secured you need to dispose of any needles and monitor the patient for changes in their condition.

Intraosseous Infusion

The use of IO access has gained acceptance over the past 15 years, but the technique has been used since the 1930s. It lost its popularity to the plastic intravenous catheters but saw a revival in the 1980s because numerous studies demonstrated the efficacy of IO administration of emergency medications in patients needing resuscitation in whom establishing intravenous (IV) access is difficult.

Historically, IO use was recommended only in children younger than 6 years. However, current guidelines for cardiopulmonary resuscitation support and battlefield trauma the use of IO techniques in patients of all ages.

Successful use in adults has been reported. IO access requires less skill and practice than central line and umbilical line placement. IO techniques have fewer serious complications than central lines and can be performed much faster than central or peripheral lines when vascular collapse is present

For patients in respiratory failure or shock, securing vascular access is crucial, along with establishing an airway and ensuring adequacy of breathing and ventilation.

Peripheral intravenous catheter insertion is often difficult, if not impossible, in patients circulatory collapse due to shock, especially children and infants.

Intraosseous (IO) needle placement, shown in the images below, provides a route for administering fluid, blood, and medication. An IO line is as efficient as an intravenous route and can be inserted quickly, even in the most poorly perfused patients.

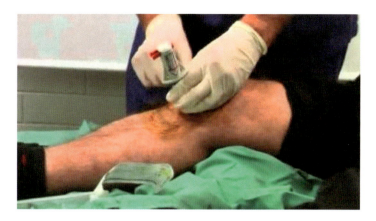

The risks and complications of Intraosseous (IO) insertion are few, and the benefits far outweigh the risks in a trauma patient without intravenous (IV) access who needs rapid administration of medication or fluid.

Extravasation of fluid is the most common complication. It typically occurs when a needle is misplaced. Rarely, extravasation occurs with a properly placed needle and is associated with excessive movement during or after insertion, which may lead to enlargement of the entry site in the bone relative to the diameter of the needle.

Starting an IO Line

You will need the following equipment and supplies:

- Alcohol swabs
- Intraosseous needles and/or IO Gun (shown below)
- IV administration set
- IV solution

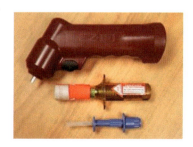

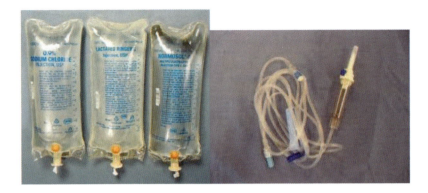

The most common site recommended for Intraosseous (IO) insertion is the proximal tibia because it provides a flat surface with a thin layer of overlying tissue and ease of identifying landmarks. Also, it is distant from the airway and chest, where resuscitation attempts are in progress. The procedure for IO insertion in the proximal tibia is as follows:

NOTE: The site of choice for Intraosseous infusion is the superior portion of the tibia, 1-2 finger widths below the tibial tuberosity in children under age 6. The single recommended site of insertion for adults is the manubrium (top 1/3 of the sternum), or on the midline and 1.5 cm (5/8 inch) below the sternal notch.

- Identify the tibial tuberosity, just below the knee, by palpation.
- Locate a consistent flat area of bone 2 cm distal and slightly medial to the tibial tuberosity. (Identifying these landmarks helps avoid hitting the growth plate.)

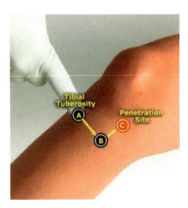

- Support the flexed knee by placing a towel under the calf.

- If time permits, cleanse the area with an iodine solution and drape it. Perform insertion using sterile gloves and technique.
- Inject local anesthetic (1% lidocaine, if available) into the skin, into the subcutaneous tissue, and over the periosteum, especially if the patient is awake and time permits.
- Insert the IO needle through the skin and subcutaneous tissue; this should occur easily. Upon reaching the bone, hold the needle with the index finger and thumb as close to the entry point as possible and, with constant pressure on the needle with the palm of the same hand, use a twisting motion to advance the needle through the cortex until reaching the marrow. A 10-15° caudal angulation may be used to further decrease the risk of hitting the growth plate, but direct entry parallel to the bone is acceptable.
- Advance the needle from the cortex into the marrow space, at which point a popping sensation or lack of resistance is felt. Do not advance the needle any farther.
- The first indication of proper placement occurs when the needle stands up on its own. At this point, remove the inner trocar, attach a syringe to the needle, and aspirate bone marrow. Obtaining marrow confirms placement.
- If marrow is not aspirated, push a 5-mL to 10-mL bolus of isotonic sodium chloride solution through the syringe. Resistance to flow should be minimal, and extravasation should not be evident. Observing the calf area is important.
- If flow is good and extravasation is not evident, connect the intravenous (IV) line with a 3-way stopcock at the needle, and secure the needle with gauze pads and tape.

Although fluid may run from the IV line by gravity, the rate is too slow for resuscitation. Faster rates of infusion occur by drawing up 30-mL to 60-mLfrom the IV bag and administering manual fluid boluses via the stopcock.

Administering medications this way is much easier, as well, and it provides more accurate administration of fluid to small infants and children. As an alternative for larger boluses, pressure bag or BP cuff wrapped around the IV bag can be used to increase flow.

The only absolute reason for not using IO is fracture of the tibia or long bones, which are potential sites for Intraosseous (IO) insertion.

Saphenous Vein Cutdown

Timely establishment of vascular access is a critical component of the care of the acutely ill or injured patient. Peripheral venous cutdown, once a mainstay in the care of the severely traumatized patient, has progressively lost favor since the introduction of the Seldinger technique of central venous line placement.

In fact, recent editions of the Advanced Trauma Life Support (ATLS) text refer to saphenous venous cutdown as an optional skill to be taught at the discretion of the instructor. In certain patients, percutaneous vascular access may be impossible to achieve or result in unacceptable time delays. In these situations, the ability to rapidly and proficiently perform peripheral venous cutdown techniques may prove invaluable and potentially lifesaving.

A saphenous vein cutdown should only be used when all other means of vascular access have failed since it is potentially life threatening if it is not performed correctly.

Equipment

- Gauze pads
- Syringe, 5 mL, with a 25-gauge (ga) needle
- IV tubing
- IV Fluid
- Scalpel, No. 10 or No. 11 blade (a No. 11 X-Acto blade can be used; sterilize first)
- Curved hemostat
- Scissors
- Intravenous catheter (14 ga)
- Intravenous tubing
- Two silk ties, 3-0
- Nylon suture, 4-0, on a cutting needle
- Tourniquet (optional)

Anatomy

The greater, or long, saphenous vein, which is the longest vein in the body, originates at the ankle as a continuation of the medial marginal vein of the foot and ends at the femoral vein within the femoral triangle.

At the ankle, it crosses 1 cm anterior to the medial malleolus and continues up the anteromedial aspect of the lower leg. It continues its superficial course and lies on the posteromedial aspect at the level of the knee. In the thigh, the greater saphenous vein courses anterolaterally through the fossa ovalis, where it joins the femoral vein approximately 4 cm below the inguinal ligament. See the image below.

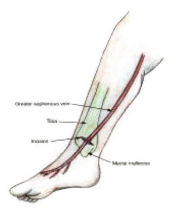

The lesser saphenous vein, also known as the short saphenous vein, does not directly anastomose with the greater saphenous vein. It begins at the lateral aspect of the ankle and runs up the posterolateral lower leg to join the popliteal vein in the popliteal fossa.

Position the patient supine with the foot externally rotated (see the illustration on the next page).

A tourniquet can be placed above the ankle but is not necessary.

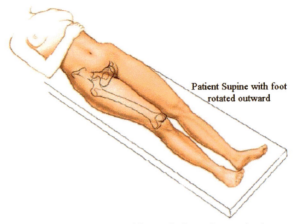
Patient Supine with foot rotated outward

- Prepare the skin of the ankle with Betadine solution and drape the area.
- Locate the vein 1 cm anterior and 1 cm superior to the medial malleolus.
- Anesthetize the skin over the area with 1% lidocaine with or without epinephrine and a 25-gauge needle.
- Make a 2.5-cm, full-thickness transverse skin incision over the site.
- With the curved hemostat, bluntly dissect the subcutaneous tissue parallel to the course of the saphenous vein.
- Free the vein from its bed for a length of 2 cm.
- With the curved hemostat, pass the ties underneath the exposed vein proximally and distally.
- Ligate the distal exposed vein and leave the free ends of the tie in place for traction.
- Pull traction on the proximal tie to further expose the vessel from its bed.
- With the scalpel, perform a small transverse venotomy through no more than 50% of the total diameter of the vessel. Be extremely careful to not fully transect the vein.
- Introduce the plastic catheter ($\geq$14 ga) through the venotomy opening, and secure it with the proximal tie.
- Attach intravenous tubing to the catheter, and close the incision with simple interrupted sutures.
- Apply sterile dressing.

(See illustrations on the next page)

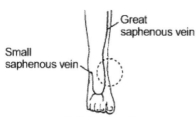 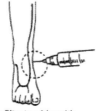

A. Palpate and locate vein

B. Infiltrate skin with local anaesthetic

 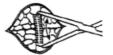

C. Make a 2 cm transverse incision

D. Expose the vein

E. Insert sutures loosely at proximal and distal end of vein

  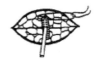

F. Make small incision in vein

G. Expose the vein and insert cannula

H. Tie upper suture to secure cannula

I. Close the wound

J. Secure cannula with suture

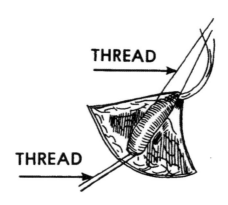

Intravenous tubing can be inserted directly into the vein for more rapid flow rates. The distal tubing can be cut on a bevel for easier insertion into the opened vein.

The opening of the venotomy site may be difficult to access. Try using a 20-ga needle bent at a right angle as a vein elevator or dilator.

Some of the complications from a saphenous vein cutdown are:

- Failed cannulation; You don't get the catheter or IV tubing into the vein
- Creation of a false passageway in the vessel wall; You don't cut fully into the vein and only create an opening in the extreme outer wall of the vein
- Hemorrhage
- Air embolus; The rapid entry of large volumes of air (>0.30 mL/kg/min) into the venous circulatory system can overwhelm the air-filtering capacity of the pulmonary vessels, resulting in a myriad of cellular changes. The air embolism effects on the pulmonary vasculature can lead to serious inflammatory changes in the pulmonary vessels; these include direct endothelial damage and accumulation of platelets, fibrin, neutrophils, and lipid droplets
- Venous thrombosis
- Infection
- Nerve transection
- Artery transection

All of these can be potentially life threatening so take all due precautions while performing a saphenous vein cutdown to avoid further injury or death to the patient.

6 SMALL WOUND CARE

Wound Debridement

When dead tissue (necrotic) or foreign material is present in a wound, sharp or surgical debridement can reduce the risk of infection and sepsis and aid wound healing.

The term debridement comes from the French desbrider, meaning to unbridle. It was probably first used as a medical term by surgeons working several hundred years ago in war zones, who recognized that grossly contaminated soft tissue wounds had a better chance of healing (and the soldier surviving) if the affected tissue was surgically removed to reveal a healthy bleeding wound surface.

A modern definition for such sharp methods of debridement is the removal of dead or necrotic tissue or foreign material from and around a wound to expose healthy tissue using a sterile scalpel, scissors or both. It can be performed as a surgical procedure in the operating theatre, involving extensive and aggressive removal of tissue with or without general anesthesia (surgical debridement), or be more conservative, involving repeated minor tissue sparing debridement that can be performed at the bedside or in a procedure room (sharp debridement).

Although surgical debridement is rapid and can involve the removal of large volumes of tissue at one time, sharp debridement should be considered as the gold standard as it can reduce the risk of wound complications and aid the healing process.

An ulcer or open wound cannot be properly assessed until all the devitalized tissue is removed. Dead or foreign material in a wound also adds to the risk of infection and sepsis and inhibits wound healing. A number of mechanisms are involved:
- Dead tissue acts as a medium for bacterial growth, particularly anaerobes such as Bacteroides species and gas gangrene caused by *Clostridium perfringens* in military surgical practice
- Excessive inflammatory response, which results from the presence of necrotic or foreign material, adds to the systemic release of cytokines such as tumor necrosis factor and interleukins which promote a septic response
- Necrotic tissues retard wound contraction, the principle contribution to wound closure when wounds are left to heal by secondary intention.

It can sometimes be difficult to determine whether the tissue covering a wound is physiological, such as a scab, or a pathological eschar, which is having a negative impact on healing. Attempts to aid clinical recognition have included the injection of supravital dyes, tissue oximetry, Doppler techniques, and even biopsy. Gangrenous, necrotic, ischemic and devitalized tissue all need to be removed by debridement.

Careful assessment is essential before taking the decision to debride a wound, particularly as there are some instances when necrotic tissue should be left alone.

For example, when there is underlying vascular disease with associated gangrene it is conventional to wait for a line of demarcation. The degree of underlying ischemia should be assessed and corrective vascular surgery considered.

It is also possible that necrotic material may auto-amputate itself. Early intervention can precipitate wet infected gangrene which spreads proximally and may need an urgent higher amputation.

Methods of Debridement

- **Surgical and sharp-** using scalpel and scissors. Highly selective with rapid results. Should only be undertaken by a skilled practitioner.

- **Mechanical-** such as hydrotherapy and wound irrigation. Rehydration can ease removal of the surface eschar and removes surface debris. However, these are relatively slow techniques and there is little evidence to support their use. Potential for cross infection needs to be considered if using hydrotherapy. There is also a theoretical risk of fluid embolism and promotion of infection if irrigation is too vigorous.

- **Maggot Therapy-** In maggot therapy, a number of small maggots are introduced to a wound in order to consume necrotic tissue, and do so far more precisely than is possible in a normal surgical operation. Larvae of the green bottle fly are used, which primarily feed on the necrotic (dead) tissue of the living host without attacking living tissue. Maggots can debride a wound in a day or two. The maggots derive nutrients through a process known as "extracorporeal digestion" by secreting a broad spectrum of proteolytic enzymes that liquefy necrotic tissue, and absorb the semi-liquid result within a few days. In an optimum wound environment maggots molt twice, increasing in length from 1–2 mm to 8–10 mm, and in girth, within a period of 3–4 days by ingesting necrotic tissue, leaving a clean wound free of necrotic tissue when they are removed. When they stay longer or too many are used, healthy tissue is removed as well.

Once the decision has been made to close a wound it must be debrided to aid in healing and to reduce the risk of infection. The use of sharp debridement AND hydrotherapy (irrigation) together will greatly speed the process.

Determining what tissue must be removed is based upon identifying what tissue has been compromised and which has not. Guideline is determining tissue viability are color, consistency, and the ability to bleed.

Viable tissue will be reddish in color, firm in consistency, and have an adequate blood supply. Healthy muscle tissue will contract when cut. Often debridement can be restricted to a narrow edge around the wound.

Unlike skin, muscle must be removed aggressively. Dead muscle tissue is near perfect medium for gaseous gangrene. Any damaged, bruised, or non-contracting muscle tissue MUST be removed COMPLETELY and all pockets must be laid open and "saucered" so the wound can drain freely.

In conjunction with debridement aggressive irrigation should be used as well. Irrigation of the wound removes contaminates from the wound and helps keep the tissues moist. A 60 cc syringe can be used in the field for wound irrigation.

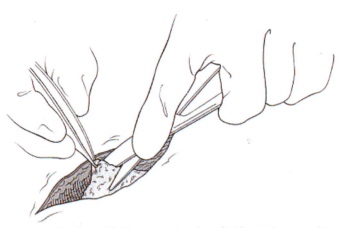

Technique to débride deep dermis and superficial fascia (subcutaneous fat).

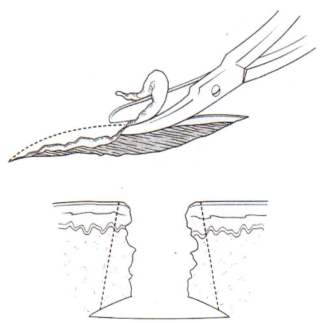

Technique for excision by careful tissue scissor trimming of devitalized epidermis and dermis. Note the angle of excision, which facilitates wound-edge eversion during percutaneous closure.

    The pictures on the following pages show the foot of an Afghani Truck driver who the beginning of a diabetic ulcer on his foot that had become infected and I had to debride.

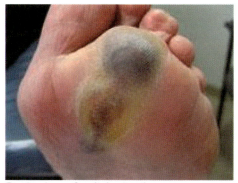
Beginning of a diabetic ulcer

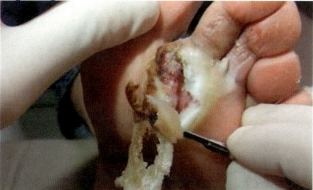
Debriding the ulcer

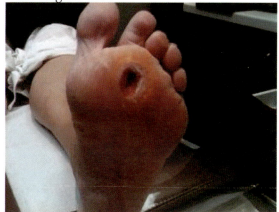
After debridement

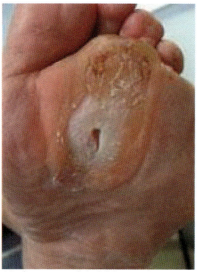
10 days post debridement

The wound required debridement two more times before it healed completely.

Suturing

As a method for closing cutaneous wounds, the technique of suturing is thousands of years old. Although suture materials and aspects of the technique have changed, the goals remain the same: closing dead space, supporting and strengthening wounds until healing increases their tensile strength, approximating skin edges for an aesthetically pleasing and functional result, and minimizing the risks of bleeding and infection.

Proper suturing technique is needed to ensure good results in dermatologic surgery. The postoperative appearance of a beautifully designed closure or flap can be compromised if an incorrect suture technique is chosen or if the execution is poor. Conversely, meticulous suturing technique cannot fully compensate for improper surgical technique. Poor incision placement with respect to relaxed skin tension lines, excessive removal of tissue, or inadequate undermining may limit the surgeon's options in wound closure and suture placement. Gentle handling of the tissue is also important to optimize wound healing.

The choice of suture technique depends on the type and anatomic location of the wound, the thickness of the skin, the degree of tension, and the desired cosmetic result. The proper placement of sutures enhances the precise approximation of the wound edges, which helps minimize and redistribute skin tension.

Wound eversion is essential to maximize the likelihood of good epidermal approximation. Eversion is desirable to minimize the risk of scar depression secondary to tissue contraction during healing.

Usually, inversion is not desirable, and it probably does not decrease the risk of hypertrophic scarring in an individual with a propensity for hypertrophic scars. The elimination of dead space, the restoration of natural anatomic contours, and the minimization of suture marks are also important to optimize the cosmetic and functional results.

The techniques of suture placement for each type of stitch will be described, the rationale for choosing one suture technique over another are reviewed, and the advantages and disadvantages of each suture technique are discussed.

Frequently, more than one suture technique is needed for optimal closure of a wound. After reading this chapter you should have an understanding of how and why particular sutures are chosen and an appreciation of the basic methods of placing each type of suture.

Basic suturing principles

Many varieties of suture material and needles are available to you. The choice of sutures and needles is determined by the location of the laceration or lesion, the thickness of the skin in that location, and the amount of tension exerted on the wound.

Regardless of the specific suture and needle chosen, the basic techniques of needle holding, needle driving, and knot placement remain the same.

Needle construction

- The needle has 3 sections. The point is the sharpest portion and is used to penetrate the tissue. The body represents the mid portion of the needle. The swage is the thickest portion of the needle and the portion to which the suture material is attached.
- In cutaneous surgery, 2 main types of needles are used: cutting and reverse cutting. Both needles have a triangular body. A cutting needle has a sharp edge on the inner curve of the needle that is

directed toward the wound edge. A reverse cutting needle has a sharp edge on the outer curve of the needle that is directed away from the wound edge, which reduces the risk of the suture pulling through the tissue. For this reason, the reverse cutting needle is used more often than the cutting needle in cutaneous surgery (see image on the next page).

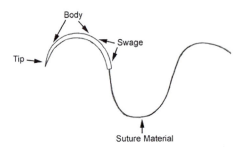

Suture placement

- A needle holder is used to grasp the needle at the distal portion of the body, one half to three quarters of the distance from the tip of the needle, depending on your preference. The needle holder is tightened by squeezing it until the first ratchet catches. The needle holder should not be tightened excessively because damage to both the needle and the needle holder may result. The needle is held vertically and longitudinally perpendicular to the needle holder (see image below).

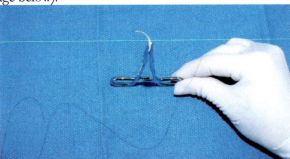

- Incorrect placement of the needle in the needle holder may result in a bent needle, difficult penetration of the skin, and/or an undesirable angle of entry into the tissue. The needle holder is held by placing the thumb and the fourth finger into the loops and by placing the index finger on the fulcrum of the needle holder to provide stability (see first image below). Alternatively, the needle holder may be held in the palm to increase dexterity (see second image on next page).

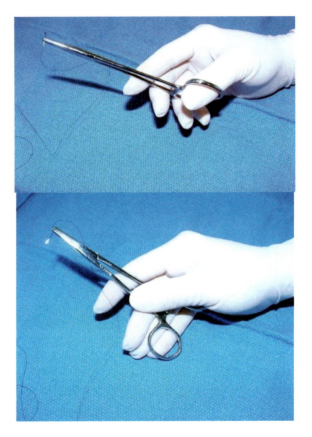

- The tissue must be stabilized to allow suture placement. Depending on the surgeon's preference, toothed or untoothed forceps or skin hooks may be used to gently grasp the tissue. Excessive trauma to the tissue being sutured should be avoided to reduce the possibility of tissue strangulation and necrosis. Forceps are necessary for grasping the needle as it exits the tissue after a pass. Prior to removing the needle holder, grasping and stabilizing the needle is important. This maneuver decreases the risk of losing the needle in

the dermis or subcutaneous fat, and it is especially important if small needles are used in areas such as the back, where large needle bites are necessary for proper tissue approximation.
- The needle should always penetrate the skin at a 90° angle, which minimizes the size of the entry wound and promotes eversion of the skin edges. The needle should be inserted 1-3 mm from the wound edge, depending on skin thickness. The depth and angle of the suture depends on the particular suturing technique. In general, the 2 sides of the suture should become mirror images, and the needle should also exit the skin perpendicular to the skin surface.

Knot tying

- Once the suture is satisfactorily placed, it must be secured with a knot. The instrument tie is used most commonly in cutaneous surgery. The square knot is traditionally used. First, the tip of the needle holder is rotated clockwise around the long end of the suture material for 2 complete turns. The tip of the needle holder is used to grasp the short end of the suture. The short end of the suture is pulled through the loops of the long end by crossing the hands, such that the 2 ends of the suture material are situated on opposite sides of the suture line. The needle holder is rotated counterclockwise once around the long end of the suture. The short end is grasped with the needle holder tip, and the short end is pulled through the loop again.
- The suture should be tightened sufficiently to approximate the wound edges without constricting the tissue. Sometimes, leaving a small loop of suture after the second throw is helpful. This reserve loop allows the stitch to expand slightly and is helpful in preventing the strangulation of tissue because the tension exerted on the suture increases with increased wound edema. Depending on the surgeon's preference, 1-2 additional throws may be added.
- Properly squaring successive ties is important. That is, each tie must be laid down perfectly parallel to the previous tie. This procedure is important in preventing the creation of a granny knot, which tends to slip and is inherently weaker than a properly squared knot. When the desired number of throws is completed, the suture material may be cut (if interrupted stitches are used), or the next suture may be placed (see image on the next page).

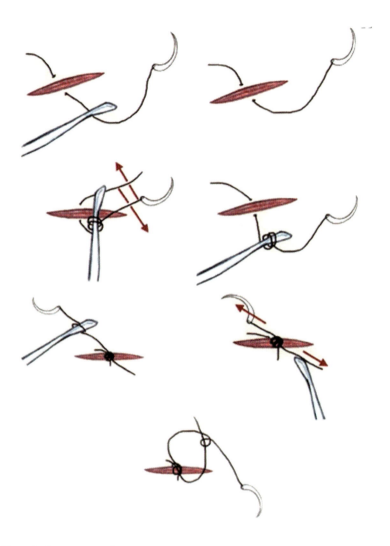

Simple interrupted sutures

- Compared with running sutures, interrupted sutures are easy to place, have greater tensile strength, and have less potential for causing wound edema and impaired cutaneous circulation. Interrupted sutures also allow the surgeon to make adjustments as needed to properly align wound edges as the wound is sutured.
- Disadvantages of interrupted sutures include the length of time required for their placement and the greater risk of

crosshatched marks (i.e., train tracks) across the suture line. The risk of crosshatching can be minimized by removing sutures early to prevent the development of suture tracks.

Simple running sutures

- Running sutures are useful for long wounds in which wound tension has been minimized with properly placed deep sutures and in which approximation of the wound edges is good. This type of suture may also be used to secure a split- or full-thickness skin graft. Theoretically, less scarring occurs with running sutures compared with interrupted sutures because fewer knots are made with simple running sutures; however, the number of needle insertions remains the same.
- Advantages of the simple running suture include quicker placement and more rapid reapproximation of wound edges, compared with simple interrupted sutures. Disadvantages include possible crosshatching, the risk of dehiscence if the suture material ruptures, difficulty in making fine adjustments along the suture line, and puckering of the suture line when the stitches are placed in thin skin.

Running locked sutures

- Locked sutures have increased tensile strength; therefore, they are useful in wounds under moderate tension or in those requiring additional hemostasis because of oozing from the skin edges.
- Running locked sutures have an increased risk of impairing the microcirculation surrounding the wound, and they can cause tissue strangulation if placed too tightly. Therefore, this type of suture should be used only in areas with good vascularization. In particular, the running locked suture may be useful on the scalp or in the postauricular sulcus, especially when additional hemostasis is needed.

Vertical mattress sutures

- A vertical mattress suture is especially useful in maximizing wound eversion, reducing dead space, and minimizing tension across the wound. One of the disadvantages of this suture is crosshatching. The risk of crosshatching is greater because of increased tension across the wound and the 4 entry and exit points of the stitch in the skin.

- The recommended time for removal of this suture is 5-7 days (before formation of epithelial suture tracks is complete) to reduce the risk of scarring. If the suture must be left in place longer, bolsters may be placed between the suture and the skin to minimize contact. The use of bolsters minimizes strangulation of the tissues when the wound swells in response to postoperative edema. Placing each stitch precisely and taking symmetric bites is especially important with this suture.

Half-buried vertical mattress sutures

- The half-buried vertical mattress is used in cosmetically important areas such as the face.

Pulley sutures

- The pulley suture facilitates greater stretching of the wound edges and is used when additional wound closure strength is desired.

Far-near near-far modified vertical mattress sutures

- The pulley suture is useful when tissue expansion is desired, and it may be used intraoperatively for this purpose. The suture is also useful when beginning the closure of a wound that is under significant tension. By placing pulley stitches first, the wound edges can be approximated, thereby facilitating the placement of buried sutures.
- When wound closure is complete, the pulley stitches may be either left in place or removed if wound tension has been adequately distributed after placement of the buried and surface sutures.

Horizontal mattress suture

- The horizontal mattress suture is useful for wounds under high tension because it provides strength and wound

eversion. This suture may also be used as a stay stitch to temporarily approximate wound edges, allowing placement of simple interrupted or subcuticular stitches. The temporary stitches are removed after the tension is evenly distributed across the wound.
- Horizontal mattress sutures may be left in place for a few days if wound tension persists after placement of the remaining stitches. In areas of extremely high tension at risk for dehiscence, horizontal mattress sutures may be left in place even after removal of the superficial skin sutures. However, they have a high risk of producing suture marks if left in place for longer than 7 days.
- Horizontal mattress sutures may be placed prior to a proposed excision as a skin expansion technique to reduce tension. Improved eversion may be achieved with this stitch in wounds without significant tension by using small bites and a fine suture.
- In addition to the risk of suture marks, horizontal sutures have a high risk of tissue strangulation and wound edge necrosis if tied too tightly. Taking generous bites, using bolsters, and cinching the suture only as tightly as necessary to approximate the wound edges may decrease the risk, as does removing the sutures as early as possible. Placing sutures at a greater distance from the wound edge facilitates their removal.

Half-buried horizontal sutures or tip stitches or 3-point corner stitches

- The half-buried horizontal suture or tip stitch is used primarily to position the corners and tips of flaps and to perform M-plasties and V-Y closures. The corner stitch may provide increased blood flow to flap tips, lowering the risk of necrosis and improving aesthetic outcomes. However, in larger flaps with greater tension, this technique has been reported to position the flap tip deeper than the surrounding tissue, often resulting in a depressed scar.

Absorbable buried sutures

- Absorbable buried sutures are used as part of a layered closure in wounds under moderate-to-high tension. Buried sutures provide support to the wound and reduce tension on the wound edges, allowing better epidermal approximation of the wound. They are also used to eliminate dead space, or they are used as anchor sutures to fix the overlying tissue to the underlying structures.

Dermal-subdermal sutures

- A buried dermal-subdermal suture maximizes wound eversion. It is placed so that the suture is more superficial away from the wound edge.

Buried horizontal mattress suture

- The buried horizontal mattress suture is used to eliminate dead space, reduce the size of a defect, or reduce tension across wounds.

Running horizontal mattress sutures

- The running horizontal mattress suture is used for skin eversion. It is useful in areas with a high tendency for inversion, such as the neck. It can also be useful for reducing the spread of facial scars. If the sutures are tied too tightly, tissue strangulation is a risk. While slightly more time consuming, this technique appears to result in smoother and flatter scars as compared to simple running sutures.

Running subcuticular sutures

- The running subcuticular suture is valuable in areas in which the tension is minimal, the dead space has been eliminated, and the best possible cosmetic result is desired. Because the epidermis is penetrated only at the beginning and end of the suture line, the subcuticular suture effectively eliminates the risk of crosshatching.
- The suture does not provide significant wound strength, although it does precisely approximate the wound edges. Therefore, the running subcuticular suture is best reserved for wounds in which the tension has been eliminated with deep sutures, and the wound edges are of approximately equal thicknesses.

Running subcutaneous sutures

- The running subcutaneous suture is used to close the deep portion of surgical defects under moderate tension. It is used in place of buried dermal sutures in large wounds when a quick closure is desired. Disadvantages of running subcutaneous sutures include the risk of suture breakage and the formation of dead space beneath the skin surface.

Running subcutaneous corset plication stitches

- The corset plication technique is used in wounds wider than 4 cm that are under excess tension. This suture creates natural eversion and better wound edge approximation. Placement of this stitch eases subsequent placement of intradermal sutures, as wound diameter and tension are reduced significantly. Strength of the suture relies on inclusion of the septations from the fascial layer beneath the subcutaneous tissue. If tissue ruptured postoperatively, tension would be distributed more broadly. Potential problems include suture breakage and wound distortion.

Modified half-buried horizontal mattress sutures

- The modified corner stitch allows for equal eversion of the flap tip edges and improved aesthetic outcomes. While it may increase risk of necrosis if tied too tightly, the incidence of flap tip necrosis was found to be comparable with that of the traditional corner stitch.

Deep tip stitch

- This stitch is used for M-plasty, W-plasty flaps, and V-Y closures to increase wound eversion. It provides longer-term support to the flap than the traditional corner stitch and improves alignment of the tip with the sides of closure. This technique also avoids surface sutures, decreasing the risk of track marks. Flap tip necrosis and complications were comparable to that of standard sutures.

Equipment

- Needle
- Needle holder
- Suture material

Simple interrupted sutures

- The most commonly used and versatile suture in cutaneous surgery is the simple interrupted suture. This suture is placed by inserting the needle perpendicular to the epidermis, traversing the epidermis and the full thickness of the dermis, and exiting perpendicular to the epidermis on the opposite side of the wound. The 2 sides of the stitch should be symmetrically placed in terms of depth and width. In general, the suture should have a flask-shaped configuration, that is, the stitch should be wider at its base (dermal side) than at its superficial portion (epidermal side). If the stitch encompasses a greater volume of tissue at the base than at its apex, the resulting compression at the base forces the tissue upward and promotes eversion of the wound edges. This maneuver decreases the likelihood of creating a depressed scar as the wound retracts during healing (see image below).

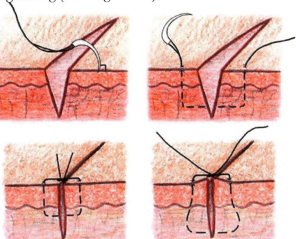

In general, tissue bites should be evenly placed so that the wound edges meet at the same level to minimize the possibility of mismatched wound-edge heights (i.e., stepping).

However, the size of the bite taken from the 2 sides of the wound can be deliberately varied by modifying the distance of the needle insertion site from the wound edge, the distance of the needle exit site from the wound edge, and the depth of the bite taken.

The use of differently sized needle bites on each side of the wound can correct preexisting asymmetry in edge thickness or height. Small bites can be used to precisely coapt wound edges.

Large bites can be used to reduce wound tension. Proper tension is important to ensure precise wound approximation while preventing tissue strangulation. The image below shows a line of interrupted sutures.

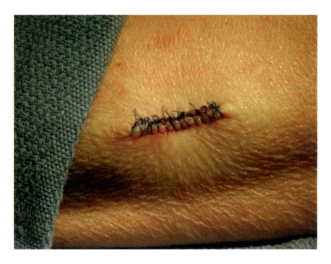

Simple running sutures

- The simple running suture is an uninterrupted series of simple interrupted sutures. The suture is started by placing a simple interrupted stitch, which is tied but not cut. A series of simple sutures are placed in succession without tying or cutting the suture material after each pass. Sutures should be evenly spaced, and tension should be evenly distributed along the suture line. The line of stitches is completed by tying a knot after the last pass at the end of the suture line. The knot is tied between the tail end of the suture material where it exits the wound and the loop of the last suture placed. The image below shows a running suture line.

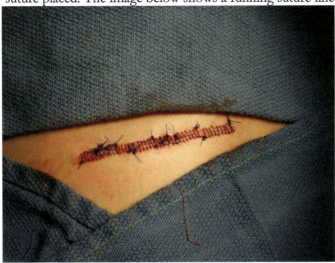

Running locked sutures

- The simple running suture may be locked or left unlocked. The first knot of a running locked suture is tied as in a traditional running suture and may be locked by passing the needle through the loop preceding it as each stitch is placed. This suture is also known as the baseball stitch (see image below) because of the final appearance of the running locked suture line.

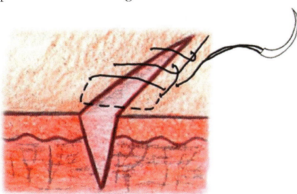

Vertical mattress sutures

- The vertical mattress suture is a variation of the simple interrupted suture. It consists of a simple interrupted stitch placed wide and deep into the wound edge and a second more superficial interrupted stitch placed closer to the wound edge and in the opposite direction. The width of the stitch should be increased in proportion to the amount of tension on the wound. That is, the higher the tension, the wider the stitch (see image below).

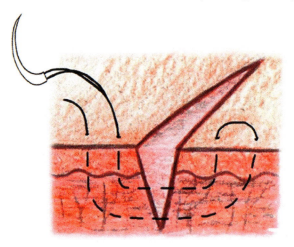

Half-buried vertical mattress sutures

- The half-buried vertical mattress suture is a modification of the vertical mattress suture and eliminates 2 of the 4 entry points, thereby reducing scarring. The half-buried vertical mattress suture is placed in the same manner as the vertical mattress suture, except that the needle penetrates the skin to the level of the deep part of the dermis on one side of the wound, takes a bite in the deep part of the dermis on the opposite side of the wound without exiting the skin, crosses back to the original side of the wound, and exits the skin. Entry and exit points therefore are kept on one side of the wound.

Pulley sutures

- The pulley suture is a modification of the vertical mattress suture. When pulley sutures are used, a vertical mattress suture is placed, the knot is left untied, and the suture is looped through the external loop on the other side of the incision and pulled across. At this point, the knot is tied. This new loop functions as a pulley, directing tension away from the other strands (see image below).

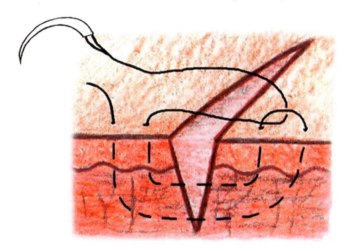

Far-near near-far modified vertical mattress sutures

- Another stitch that serves the same function as the pulley suture is the far-near near-far modification of the vertical mattress suture. The first loop is placed approximately 4-6 mm from the wound edge on the far side and approximately 2 mm from the wound edge on the near side. The suture crosses the suture line and reenters the skin on the original side at 2 mm from the wound edge on the near side. The loop is completed, and the suture exits the skin on the opposite side 4-6 mm away from the wound edge on the far side. This placement creates a pulley effect (see image on next page).

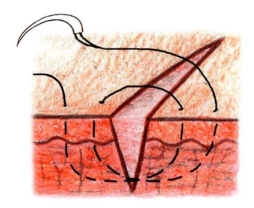

Horizontal mattress suture

- The horizontal mattress suture is placed by entering the skin 5 mm to 1 cm from the wound edge. The suture is passed deep in the dermis to the opposite side of the suture line and exits the skin equidistant from the wound edge (in effect, a deep simple interrupted stitch). The needle reenters the skin on the same side of the suture line 5 mm to 1 cm lateral of the exit point. The stitch is passed deep to the opposite side of the wound where it exits the skin and the knot is tied (see image below).

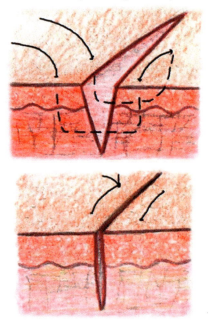

Half-buried horizontal sutures or tip stitches or 3-point corner stitches

- The half-buried horizontal suture or tip stitch begins on the side of the wound on which the flap is to be attached. The suture is passed through the dermis of the wound edge to the dermis of the flap tip. The needle is passed laterally in the same dermal plane of the flap tip, exits the flap tip, and reenters the skin to which the flap is to be attached. The needle is directed perpendicularly and exits the skin; then, the knot is tied (see image below).

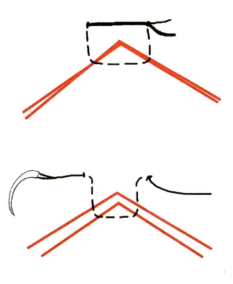

Dermal-subdermal sutures

- The suture is placed by inserting the needle parallel to the epidermis at the junction of the dermis and the subcutis. The needle curves upward and exits in the papillary dermis, again parallel to the epidermis. The needle is inserted parallel to the epidermis in the papillary dermis on the opposing edge of the wound, curves down through the reticular dermis, and exits at the base of the wound at the interface between the dermis and the subcutis and parallel to the epidermis. The knot is tied at the base of the wound to minimize the possibility of tissue reaction and extrusion of the knot. If the suture is placed more superficially in the dermis at 2-4 mm from the wound edge, eversion is increased.

Buried horizontal mattress suture

- The buried horizontal mattress suture is a purse-string suture. The suture must be placed in the mid-to-deep part of the dermis to prevent the skin from tearing. If tied too tightly, the suture may strangulate the approximated tissue.

Running horizontal mattress sutures

- A simple suture is placed, and the knot is tied but not cut. A continuous series of horizontal mattress sutures is placed, with the final loop tied to the free end of the suture material.

Running subcuticular sutures

- The running subcuticular suture is a buried form of the running horizontal mattress suture. It is placed by taking horizontal bites through the papillary dermis on alternating sides of the wound. No suture marks are visible, and the suture may be left in place for several weeks (see image below).

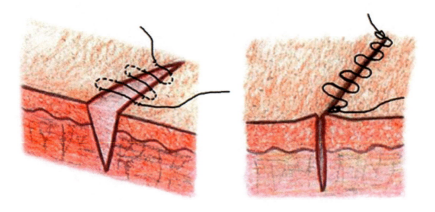

Running subcutaneous sutures

- The running subcutaneous suture begins with a simple interrupted subcutaneous suture, which is tied but not cut. The suture is looped through the subcutaneous tissue by successively passing through the opposite sides of the wound. The knot is tied at the opposite end of the wound by knotting the long end of the suture material to the loop of the last pass that was placed.

Running subcutaneous corset plication stitches

- Before inserting the needle, forceps are used to pull firmly on at least 1-2 cm of tissue to ensure tissue strength. The corset plication includes at least 1-2 cm of adipose tissue and fascia within each bite. After the first bite is tied, bites are taken on opposite sides of the wound in a running fashion along the defect. The free end is pulled firmly reducing the size of the defect, and the suture is then tied.

Variations of tip (corner) sutures

Modified half-buried horizontal mattress sutures

- This stitch places an additional vertical mattress suture superficial to the half-buried horizontal mattress suture. A small skin hook instead of forceps is used to avoid trauma of the flap.

Deep tip stitch

- The deep tip stitch is essentially a full-buried form of the 3-corner stitch. The suture is placed into the deep dermis of the wound edge to which the flap is to be attached, passed through the dermis of the flap tip, and inserted into the deep dermis of the opposite wound edge.

Knot Tying

Now that you have decided on which sutres technique you are going to use to close the wound you will need to secure those sutures by tying a knot. When tying off your sutures remember, "Approximate, Don't strangulate!" You want to bring the two sides of the wound together NOT squeeze the life out of them, bring your knot to the skin, not the skin to your knot.

There are many knot tying variations and techniques, all with the intention of completing a secure, square knot. A complete square knot consists of two sequential throws that lie in opposite directions. This is necessary to create a knot that will not slip.

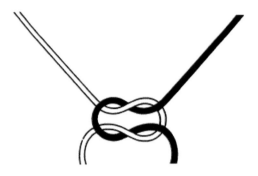

Surgeons knot

A surgeon's knot is a variation in which a double throw is followed by a single throw to increase the friction on the suture material and to decrease the initial slip until a full square knot has been completed.

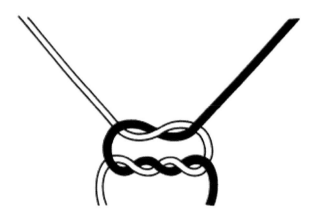

Use a minimum of two complete square knots on any substantive vessel and more when using monofilament suture. If the suture material is slippery, more knot throws will be required to ensure that the suture does not come undone or slip. When using a relatively "non-slippery" material such as silk, as few as three throws may be sufficient to ensure a secure knot.

Cut sutures of slippery materials longer than those of "non-slippery" materials. There is a balance between the need for security of the knot and the desire to leave as little foreign material in the wound as possible.

Suture Tying Techniques

There are three basic techniques of knot tying and they are:

Instrument Tie

This is the most straightforward and the most commonly used technique; take care to ensure that the knots are tied correctly.

You must cross your hands to produce a square knot; to prevent slipping, use a surgeon's knot on the first throw only.

Do not use instrument ties if the patient's life depends on the security of the knot.

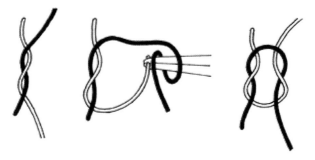

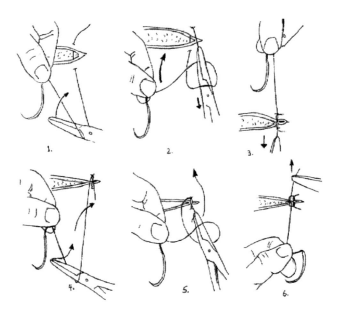

One Handed Knot

Use the one handed technique to place deep seated knots and when one limb of the suture is immobilized by a needle or instrument.

Hand tying has the advantage of tactile sensations lost when using instruments; if you place the first throw of the knot twice, it will slide into place, but will have enough friction to hold while the next throw is placed.

This is an alternative to the surgeon's knot, but must be followed with a square knot.

To attain a square knot, the limbs of the suture must be crossed even when the knot is placed deeply.

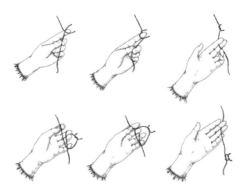

Two Handed Knot

The two handed knot is the most secure. Both limbs of the suture are moved during its placement. A surgeon's knot is easily formed using a two handed technique.

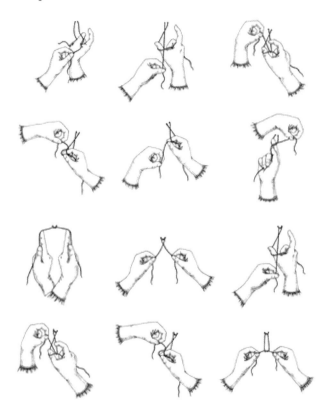

Suture removal

- Sutures should be removed within 1-2 weeks of their placement, depending on the anatomic location. Prompt removal reduces the risk of suture marks, infection, and tissue reaction. The average wound usually achieves approximately 8% of its expected tensile strength 1-2 weeks after surgery. To prevent dehiscence and spread of the scar, sutures should not be removed too soon.
- As a general rule, the greater the tension across a wound, the longer the sutures should remain in place. As a guide, on the face, sutures should be removed in 5-7 days; on the neck, 7 days; on the scalp, 10 days; on the trunk and upper extremities, 10-14 days; and on the

lower extremities, 14-21 days. Sutures in wounds under greater tension may need to be left in place slightly longer. Buried sutures, which are placed with absorbable suture material, are left in place because they dissolve.
- Proper suture removal technique is important to maintain good results after sutures are properly selected and executed. Sutures should be gently elevated with forceps, and one side of the suture should be cut. Then, the suture is gently grasped by the knot and gently pulled toward the wound or suture line until the suture material is completely removed. If the suture is pulled away from the suture line, the wound edges may separate. Steri-Strips may be applied with a tissue adhesive to provide continued supplemental wound support after the sutures are removed.

Alternative Methods of Wound Closure

Steri-Strips

- Wound closure tapes, or Steri-Strips, are reinforced microporous surgical adhesive tape. Steri-Strips are used to provide extra support to a suture line, either when running subcuticular sutures are used or after sutures are removed.
- Wound closure tapes may reduce spreading of the scar if they are kept in place for several weeks after suture removal. Often, they are used with a tissue adhesive. Because they have a tendency to fall off, they are used mainly in low-tension wounds and rarely for primary wound closure.

Staples

- Stainless steel staples are frequently used in wounds under high tension, including wounds on the scalp and trunk. Advantages of staples include quick placement, minimal tissue reaction, low risk of infection, and strong wound closure. Disadvantages include less precise wound edge alignment and cost.

Tissue adhesive

- Superglues that contain acrylates may be applied to superficial wounds to block pinpoint skin hemorrhages and to precisely coapt wound edges. Because of their bacteriostatic effects and easy application, they have gained increasing popularity. They have demonstrated either cosmetic equivalence or superiority to traditional sutures in various procedures, including sutureless closure of pediatric day surgeries, saphenous vein harvesting for coronary artery bypass, and blepharoplasty. The most commonly used adhesive, 2-octyl cyanoacrylate (Dermabond), has also been used as a skin bolster for suturing thin, atrophic skin. Advantages of these topical adhesives include rapid wound closure, painless application, reduced risk of needle sticks, no suture marks, and no removal. Disadvantages include increased cost and less tensile strength (compared to sutures).

- The use of tissue adhesives in dermatologic surgery is still evolving. It appears that using high viscosity 2-octyl cyanoacrylate in the repair of linear wounds after Mohs micrographic surgery results in cosmetic outcomes equivalent to those of epidermal sutures.
- Greenhill and O'Regan reported on the use of N-butyl 2-cyanoacrylate (Indermil) for closure of parotid wounds and its relationship to keloid and hypertrophic scar formation versus using sutures. Their results indicated a simpler technique and a comparable result. In a related area, Tsui and Gogolewski report on the use of microporous biodegradable polyurethane membranes, which may be useful for coverage of skin wounds, among other things.

7 INFECTED WOUND CARE

A Brief History of Infected Wound Care

The ancient Egyptians were the first civilization to have trained clinicians to treat physical ailments. Medical papyri, such as the Edwin Smith papyrus (circa 1600 BC) and the Ebers papyrus (circa 1534 BC), provided detailed information of management of disease, including wound management with the application of various potions and grease to assist healing.

The scale of wound infections is most evident in times of war and natural disaster. During the American Civil War, erysipelas (necrotizing infection of soft tissue) and tetanus accounted for over 17,000 deaths, according to an anonymous source in 1883. Because compound fractures at the time almost invariably were associated with infection, amputation was the only option, despite a 25-90% risk of amputation stump infection.

Koch (Professor of Hygiene and Microbiology, Berlin, 1843-1910) first recognized the cause of infective foci as secondary to microbial growth in his 19th century postulates. Semmelweis (Austrian obstetrician, 1818-1865) demonstrated a 5-fold reduction in puerperal sepsis by hand washing between performing postmortem examinations and entering the delivery room. Joseph Lister (Professor of Surgery, London, 1827-1912) and Louis Pasteur (French bacteriologist, 1822-1895) revolutionized the entire concept of wound infection. Lister recognized that antisepsis could prevent infection. In 1867, Lister placed carbolic acid into open fractures to sterilize the wound and to prevent sepsis and hence the need for amputation. In 1871, Lister began to use carbolic spray in the operating room to reduce contamination. However, the concept of wound suppuration persevered even among eminent surgeons, such as John Hunter, 1728-1793.

World War I (WWI) resulted in new types of wounds from high-velocity bullet and shrapnel injuries coupled with contamination by the mud from the trenches. Antoine Depage (Belgian military surgeon, 1862-1925) reintroduced wound debridement and delayed wound closure and relied on microbiological assessment of wound brushings as guidance for the timing of secondary wound closure. Alexander Fleming (microbiologist, London, 1881-1955) performed many of his bacteriological studies during WWI and is credited with the discovery of penicillin.

Penicillin first was used clinically in 1940 by Howard Florey. With the use of antibiotics, a new era in the management of wound infections commenced. Unfortunately, eradication of the infective plague affecting surgical wounds has not ended because of the insurgence of antibiotic-resistant bacterial strains and the nature of more adventurous surgical intervention in immunocompromised patients and in implant surgery.

Internationally, the frequency of wound infection is difficult to monitor because criteria for diagnosis might not be standardized. A survey sponsored by the World Health Organization demonstrated a prevalence of nosocomial infections varying from 3-21%, with wound infections accounting for 5-34% of the total. The 2002 survey report by the Nosocomial Infection National Surveillance Service (NINSS), which covers the period between October 1997 and September 2001, indicates that the incidence of hospital acquired infection related to surgical wounds in the United Kingdom is as high as 10% and costs the National Health Service in the United Kingdom approximately 1 billion pounds (1.8 billion dollars) annually.

Collated data on the incidence of wound infections probably underestimate true incidence because most wound infections occur when the patient is discharged, and these infections may be treated in the community without hospital notification.

Presentation

Surgical site infection is a difficult term to define accurately because it has a wide spectrum of possible clinical features.

The Centers for Disease Control and Prevention (CDC) have defined SSI to standardize data collection for the National Nosocomial Infections Surveillance (NNIS) program.[11, 12] SSIs are classified into incisional SSIs, which can be superficial or deep, or organ/space SSIs, which affect the rest of the body other than the body wall layers.

- Definitions of surgical site infection (see image below)

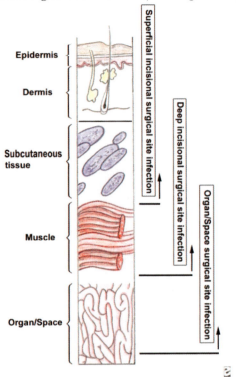

  - Superficial incisional SSI: Infection involves only skin and subcutaneous tissue of incision.
  - Deep incisional SSI: Infection involves deep tissues, such as fascial and muscle layers. This also includes infection involving both superficial and deep incision sites and organ/space SSI draining through incision.
  - Organ/space SSI: Infection involves any part of the anatomy in organs and spaces other than the incision, which was opened or manipulated during operation.
- Superficial incisional SSI is more common than deep incisional SSI and organ/space SSI. Superficial incisional SSI accounts for more than half of all SSIs for all categories of surgery. The postoperative length of stay is longer for patients with SSI, and when adjusted for other factors influencing length of stay.

According to a report by the NNIS program, wound infections are defined as follows:

- Superficial incisional SSI
    - Occurs within 30 days after the wound
    - Involves only the skin or subcutaneous tissue
    - At least 1 of the following:
        - Purulent drainage is present (culture documentation not required).
        - Organisms are isolated from fluid/tissue of the superficial incision.
        - At least 1 sign of inflammation (e.g., pain or tenderness, induration, erythema, local warmth of the wound) is present.
        - The wound is deliberately opened by the surgeon.
        - The surgeon or clinician declares the wound infected.
    - Note: A wound is not considered a superficial incisional SSI if a stitch abscess is present; if the infection is at an episiotomy, a circumcision site, or a burn wound; or if the SSI extends into fascia or muscle.
- Deep incisional SSI
    - Occurs within 30 days of the operation or within 1 year if an implant is present
    - Involves deep soft tissues (e.g., fascia and/or muscle) of the incision
    - At least 1 of the following:
        - Purulent drainage is present from the deep incision but without organ/space involvement.
        - Fascial dehiscence or fascia is deliberately separated by the surgeon because of signs of inflammation.
        - A deep abscess is identified by direct examination or during reoperation, by histopathology, or by radiologic examination.
        - The surgeon or clinician declares that a deep incisional infection is present.
- Organ/space SSI
    - Occurs within 30 days of the operation or within 1 year if an implant is present
    - Involves anatomical structures not opened or manipulated during the operation
    - At least 1 of the following:
        - Purulent drainage is present from a drain placed by a stab wound into the organ/space.
        - Organisms are isolated from the organ/space by

aseptic culturing technique.
- An abscess in the organ/space is identified by direct examination, during reoperation, or by histopathologic or radiologic examination.
- A diagnosis of organ/space SSI is made by the surgeon or clinician.

Causes

All wounds are contaminated by microbes, but in most cases, infection does not develop because innate host defenses are quite efficient in the elimination of contaminants. A complex interplay between host, microbial, and surgical factors ultimately determines the prevention or establishment of a wound infection.

- Microbiology: Microbial factors that influence the establishment of a wound infection are the bacterial inoculum, virulence, and the effect of the microenvironment. When these microbial factors are conducive, impaired host defenses set the stage for enacting the chain of events that produce wound infection.
  - Most wounds are contaminated by the patient's own endogenous flora, which are present on the skin, mucous membranes, or hollow viscera. The traditional microbial concentration quoted as being highly associated with wounds is that of bacterial counts higher than 10,000 organisms per gram of tissue (or in the case of burned sites, organisms per cm^2 of wound).
  - The usual pathogens on skin and mucosal surfaces are gram-positive cocci (notably staphylococci); however, gram-negative aerobes and anaerobic bacteria contaminate skin in the groin/perineal areas. The contaminating pathogens in gastrointestinal surgery are the multitude of intrinsic bowel flora, which include gram-negative bacilli (e.g. ,*Escherichia coli*) and gram-positive microbes, including enterococci and anaerobic organisms. See Table 1 for pathogens and their frequencies. Gram-positive organisms, particularly staphylococci and streptococci, account for most exogenous flora involved in SSIs. Sources of such pathogens include surgical/hospital personnel and intraoperative circumstances, including surgical instruments, articles brought into the operative field, and the operating room air.
  - The most common group of bacteria responsible for SSIs

are *Staphylococcus aureus*. The emergence of resistant strains has considerably increased the burden of morbidity and mortality associated with wound infections.
- Methicillin resistant *Staphylococcus aureus* (MRSA) is proving to be the scourge of modern day surgery. Like other strains of *S aureus,* MRSA can colonize the skin and body of an individual without causing sickness, and, in this way, it can be passed on to other individuals unknowingly. Problems arise in the treatment of overt infections with MRSA because antibiotic choice is very limited. MRSA infections appear to be increasing in frequency and are displaying resistance to a wider range of antibiotics.[
- Of particular concern are the vancomycin intermediate *Staphylococcus aureus* (VISA) strains of MRSA. These strains are beginning to develop resistance to vancomycin, which is currently the most effective antibiotic against MRSA. This new resistance has arisen because another species of bacteria, called enterococci, relatively commonly express vancomycin resistance.

Table 1. Pathogens Commonly Associated with Wound Infections and Frequency of Occurrence.

Pathogen	Frequency (%)
Staphylococcus aureus	20
Coagulase-negative staphylococci	14
Enterococci	12
Escherichia coli	8
Pseudomonas aeruginosa	8
Enterobacter species	7
Proteus mirabilis	3
Klebsiella pneumoniae	3
Other streptococci	3
Candida albicans	3

Group D streptococci	2
Other gram-positive aerobes	2
Bacteroides fragilis	2

Risk factors (other than microbiology)

- Decreased host resistance can be due to systemic factors affecting the patient's healing response, local wound characteristics, or operative characteristics.

- Systemic factors include age, malnutrition, hypovolemia, poor tissue perfusion, obesity, diabetes, steroids, and other immunosuppressant's.

- Wound characteristics include nonviable tissue in wound; hematoma; foreign material, including drains and sutures; dead space; poor skin preparation, including shaving; and preexistent sepsis (local or distant).

- Operative characteristics include poor surgical technique; lengthy operation (>2 h); intraoperative contamination, including infected theater staff and instruments and inadequate theater ventilation; prolonged preoperative stay in the hospital; and hypothermia.

- The type of procedure is a risk factor. Certain procedures are associated with a higher risk of wound contamination than others. Surgical wounds have been classified as clean, clean-contaminated, contaminated, and dirty-infected (see Table 2).

Table 2: Surgical Wound Classification and Subsequent Risk of Infection (If No Antibiotics Used)

Classification	Description	Infective Risk (%)
Clean (Class I)	Uninfected operative wound No acute inflammation	< 2

	Closed primarily	
	Respiratory, gastrointestinal, biliary, and urinary tracts not entered	
	No break in aseptic technique	
	Closed drainage used if necessary	
Clean-contaminated (Class II)	Elective entry into respiratory, biliary, gastrointestinal, urinary tracts and with minimal spillage	< 10
	No evidence of infection or major break in aseptic technique	
	Example: appendectomy	
Contaminated (Class III)	Nonpurulent inflammation present	About 20
	Gross spillage from gastrointestinal tract	

	Penetrating traumatic wounds < 4 hours	
	Major break in aseptic technique	
Dirty-infected (Class IV)	Purulent inflammation present	About 40
	Preoperative perforation of viscera	
	Penetrating traumatic wounds >4 hours	

Antibiotic Treatment

The use of antibiotics was a milestone in the effort to prevent wound infection. The concept of prophylactic antibiotics was established in the 1960s when experimental data established that antibiotics had to be in the circulatory system at a high enough dose at the time of incision to be effective.

General agreement exists that prophylactic antibiotics are indicated for clean-contaminated and contaminated wounds (see Table 2). Antibiotics for dirty wounds are part of the treatment because infection is established already. Clean procedures might be an issue of debate. No doubt exists regarding the use of prophylactic antibiotics in clean procedures in which prosthetic devices are inserted because infection in these cases would be disastrous for the patient. However, other clean procedures (e.g., breast surgery) may be a matter of contention.

Criteria for the use of systemic preventive antibiotics in wound care are as follows:
- Systemic preventive antibiotics should be used in the following cases:

- - A high risk of infection is associated with the mechanism of injury (e.g. stab wound, gunshot wound)
  - Consequences of infection are unusually severe (e.g., natural disaster, survival situation).
- The antibiotic should be administered as close to the time of the wound as is clinically practical. Antibiotics should be administered before induction of anesthesia in most situations.
- The antibiotic selected should have activity against the pathogens likely to be encountered in the procedure.
- Postoperative administration of preventive systemic antibiotics beyond 24 hours has not been demonstrated to reduce the risk of wound infection.

Qualities of prophylactic antibiotics include efficacy against predicted bacterial microorganisms most likely to cause infection, good tissue penetration to reach wound involved, cost effectiveness, and minimal disturbance to intrinsic body flora (e.g., gut).

The timing of administration is critically important because the concentration of the antibiotic should be at therapeutic levels at the time of debridement, during wound closure, and ideally, for a few hours after you have closed the wound. See Table 3 for specific antibiotics recommended.

The choice of antibiotic depends on 2 factors—the patient and the known or probable infecting microorganism. Patient factors include allergies, hepatic and renal function, severity of disease process, interaction with other medication(s), and age. In women, pregnancy and breastfeeding must be considered.

Table 3. Recommendations for Antibiotics

Cefotetan

Cefotetan is a second-generation cephalosporin with activity against some gram-positive cocci, gram-negative rod infections, and anaerobic bacteria. It inhibits bacterial cell wall synthesis by binding to one or more of the penicillin-binding proteins; it inhibits the final transpeptidation step of peptidoglycan synthesis, resulting in cell wall death.

Infections caused by cephalosporin- or penicillin-resistant gram-negative bacteria may respond to Cefotetan. Antibiotics have proved effective in decreasing the rate of postoperative wound infection and improving outcome in patients with intraperitoneal infection and septicemia.

Metronidazole hydrochloride (Flagyl)

Metronidazole is an imidazole ring-based antibiotic active against various anaerobic bacteria and protozoa. It is used in combination with other antimicrobial agents (except for Clostridium difficile enterocolitis).

Gentamicin sulfate

An aminoglycoside antibiotic for gram-negative coverage, gentamicin is used in combination with an agent against gram-positive organisms and one that covers anaerobes. This is not the drug of choice. Consider gentamicin if penicillin's or other less toxic drugs are contraindicated, when clinically indicated, and in mixed infections caused by susceptible staphylococci and gram-negative organisms.

Dosing regimens are numerous; adjust dose based on creatinine clearance and changes in volume of distribution. Gentamicin may be administered IV or IM.

Vancomycin hydrochloride (Vancocin)

A potent antibiotic directed against gram-positive organisms and active against enterococcal species, vancomycin is useful in the treatment of septicemia and skin-structure infections. It is indicated for patients who cannot receive or who are unresponsive to penicillin's and cephalosporin's or who have infections with resistant staphylococci.

For penetrating abdominal injuries, vancomycin is combined with an agent active against enteric flora and/or anaerobes. To avoid toxicity, the current recommendation is to assay trough levels after the third dose, with the sample drawn 0.5 h prior to next dosing. Use creatinine clearance to adjust dose in patients with renal impairment.

Vancomycin is used in conjunction with gentamicin for prophylaxis in penicillin-allergic patients undergoing GI or GU procedures.

Ampicillin sodium-sulbactam sodium (Unasyn)

This combination of a beta-lactamase inhibitor with ampicillin covers skin, enteric flora, and anaerobes. It is not ideal for nosocomial pathogens.

Veterinary Antibiotics

One question I see and hear a lot of people talk about is medicine, and their lack of factual information when it comes to antibiotics. More specifically if they can use antibiotics marketed to vets for use on animals. Most people can't convince their doctor into writing extraneous prescriptions for a SHTF scenario.

It's not a big secret that veterinary antibiotics and drugs do not require a prescription. Drugs such as Fish-MOX clearly state on their label, **"For Aquarium and Fish Use Only."** But are they really only for fish? Are these antibiotics any different than what my pharmacist gives you when your doctor writes you a prescription?

When I first started researching antibiotics for this book, all I found was information from pseudo-doctors and "scientists" from across the internet. I found nothing but conflicting information regarding the human consumption of animal antibiotics.

Many of the doctors I give credit to in the Acknowledgements of this book gave me a variety of answers or most often simply beat around the bush.

One MD would say XYZ, and another doctor would tell me ABC. Some would say that they *thought* it would be safe to use veterinarian drugs, but only in dire times or as a last resort. Others would warn against it entirely, and yet some would encourage their use in everyday applications.

Because, "The Truth is Out There", I wanted concrete information on the safety and efficacy of using animal antibiotics in humans.

As I said; Veterinary drugs ***Do Not Require a Prescription.***

That might sound more dangerous than buying pills from a Mexican street corner, but I promise you, it is not. USP-approved animal pharmaceuticals are often made in the same manufacturing plants as human pharmaceuticals and will contain the same ingredients. They are the same color, shape, and bare the same markings as human drugs. This likely boils down to cost-effectiveness for Big Pharma, but for once, is also in your interest and favor.

Let me explain. Every "drug" manufactured, sold, or brought into the United States must pass FDA regulations and is listed within the United

States Pharmacopeia, or **USP**. This is a compendium recognized officially by the Federal Food, Drug, and Cosmetic Act that contains descriptions, uses, strengths, and *standards of purity* for selected drugs and for all of their forms of dosage.

Use of the USP Verified Pharmaceutical Ingredient Mark helps ingredient manufacturers assure their customers that the quality of the ingredients they are supplying has been rigorously tested and verified by an independent authority. When the mark appears on an ingredient container or carton, it represents that USP has evaluated the ingredient and found that:

- The participant's quality system helps to ensure that the ingredient meets its label or certificate of analysis claims for identity, strength, purity, and quality.
- The ingredient has been prepared under accepted good manufacturing practices (GMP) that ensure consistency in the quality of ingredients from batch to batch.
- The ingredient meets its specifications' acceptance criteria.

So what does all of this FDA crap mean? Basically, it translates that if you see an animal drug that is labeled, "UPS Pharmaceutical grade Amoxicillin," it is the exact same pharmaceutical grade Amoxicillin that you get from Wal-Mart your doctor would prescribe you for various infections.

As for the identification or verification process, should you still feel uneasy, we can look to the FDA.

Per the Federal Food, Drug, and Cosmetic Act each capsule, tablet, or pill must be ***uniquely marked***. Two tablets with identical colors, shapes, and markings ***cannot***, by law, have different ingredients.

This is for a variety of reasons, but not limited to assisting Poison Control hotlines, hospitals, doctors, etc., in determining what someone might have ingested, overdosed on, or is causing side effects.

This picture shows the color and markings of Fish-Mox per FDA USP Guidelines.

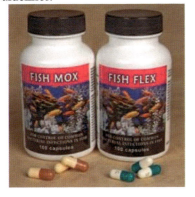

The picture below shows Amoxicillin Capsules from Wal-Mart pharmacy that I got a few months ago by prescription for an infection.

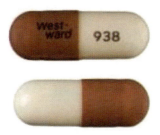

These and all antibiotics are used at specific doses for specific illnesses; the exact dosage of each and every medication is beyond the scope of this book.

Suffice it to say that most penicillin and cephalosporin (Keflex and other cephalexin) medications are taken at 500mg dosages, 3-4 times a day for adults, and 250mg dosages for children, 3-4 times a day, where Metronidazole (250mg) and Doxycycline (100mg) are taken twice a day.

It's important to have as much information as possible on medications that you plan to store for when TSHTF, so consider purchasing a hard copy of the latest Physician's Desk Reference. This book comes out yearly and has just about every bit of information that exists on a particular medication, including those that do not require prescription. Indications for use, dosage, risks, and side effects are all listed.

Sugar for infected Wounds

When sugar is applied to a wound it will normally dissolve within four hours, creating a highly concentrated environment on the wound surface. Body fluids are attracted to the wound surface to equalize the high concentration gradient (osmosis), increasing the volume of exudate produced. This appears to cleanse/irrigate the wound and to liquefy devitalized dead tissue. The dead tissue is removed each time the wound is re-dressed, promoting the generation of new tissue.

Sugar is widely used in a number of countries across Africa and there has been more limited use in the UK and the US. To date, there is scant evidence of its efficacy in infected wounds; the largest study in the US ran over a 56-month period and treated a total of 605 patients with wounds of different etiologies. The study reported rapid wound healing when using sugar and povidone-iodine to enhance wound healing.

In the UK, one small case study found that packing malodorous pressure ulcers with sugar paste stopped the odor and debrided necrotic tissue. More recently, Mphande *et al* (2007) compared the effects of sugar and honey on wound healing and observed no significant difference between the two.

The patient in the following case study is one of 21 patients who participated in a small pilot study in a UK hospital exploring the effectiveness of dry granulated sugar on exudation of wounds. This study aimed to develop a protocol for use with a randomized controlled trial to compare dry granulated sugar with standard treatment.

Sugar has been used as an infected wound dressing for over 3500 years. The use of sugar is based on its high osmolality, which draws fluid out of the wound. Reducing water in the wound inhibits the growth of bacteria. The use of sugar also aids in the debridement of necrotic tissue, while preserving viable tissue.

Granulated sugar is placed into the wound cavity in a layer 1-cm thick and covered with a thick dressing, that can be soaked in povidone iodine as well (if no allergy to iodine) to absorb fluid drawn from the wound. The sugar dressing should be changed once or twice daily or more frequently as needed (e.g., whenever "strike-through" is seen on the bandage).

During the bandage change, the wound should be liberally lavaged (washed) with warm saline or tap water. Sugar dressings may be used until granulation tissue is seen.

Once all infection is resolved, the wound may be closed or allowed to epithelize. Because a large volume of fluid can be removed from the wound, the patient's hemodynamic and hydration status must be monitored and treated accordingly. Hypovolemia and low colloid osmotic pressure are complications that may be associated with this therapy.

The picture below shows a patient with an infected wound that was treated using sugar dressings. The photo on the left shows the wound as the patient appeared in the ER. The picture on the right shows the wound after 12 days of treatment using sugar dressings.

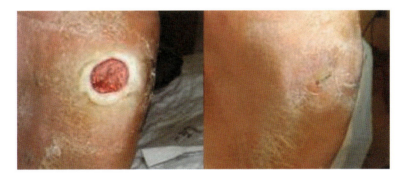

Honey Dressings

Honey has also been used for wound dressings over the centuries. Honey's beneficial effects are thought to be a result of hydrogen peroxide production from activity of the glucose oxidase enzyme. The low pH of honey also may accelerate healing.

Honey used for wound healing must be unpasteurized, and the source of the honey appears to be a factor in its effectiveness. Manuka honey may be the best option for wound care. The contact layer wound dressings should be soaked in honey before application. The bandage may be changed daily or more frequently as needed.

If we ever find ourselves without modern medical care, we will have to improvise medical strategies that we perhaps might be reluctant to consider today. Without hospitals, it will be up to **YOU** to treat infections. That responsibility will be difficult to carry out without the weapons to fight disease, such as antibiotics.

Alternative therapies should be looked at carefully, as well. Honey and garlic have known antibacterial actions, as do a number of herbs and essential oils. Be sure to integrate all medical options, traditional *and* alternative, and use every tool at your disposal to keep your community healthy.

I urge you to verify and check all medications that you order, regardless of the source, with a reputable pill identification book or website in order to make sure you truly receive what you ordered.

8 BURNS

Burns can be classified by their cause, as thermal (i.e., heat), flame, flash, contact (with a hot radiator, etc.), scald (hot water, oil, or other liquid), chemical, electric, or radiation (sunburn, x-rays, nuclear). Inhalation burn injury may occur with or without skin injury, and may be life threatening.

The depth of burn is often classified as first, second, or third degree. "Partial-thickness burns" refers to first- and second-degree burns, whereas "full-thickness burns" refers to third degree burns. A burn of 20% of the total body surface area (20% TBSA) or greater is a life-threatening burn (in the very young, very old, or those with serious medical diseases, 10% TBSA or more can be life-threatening). These patients need IV fluid resuscitation and evacuation, if possible.

Symptoms

Painful, red skin without (1st degree) or with (2nd degree) blisters; or dry, charred, non-painful skin (3rd degree), or a combination. May complain of hoarseness or coughing.

Signs

First-Degree Second-Degree Third-Degree Typical causes Sun, hot liquids, brief Hot liquids, flash or Flame, prolonged contact flash burns flame, chemical with hot liquid or hot object, electricity, chemical

Color Pink or red Pink or mottled red Dark brown, charred, pearly white, translucent with visible, thrombosed veins

Surface Dry Moist, weeping, blisters Dry and inelastic
Sensation Painful Very painful Anesthetic
Depth Epidermis and portions Epidermis, dermis, and
of the dermis possibly deep structures
Healing Few days Few weeks Skin grafting or slow inward
contraction of edges
Warning: Airway obstruction may present suddenly or gradually over a period of hours with: stridor, hoarseness, coughing, carbon in the sputum or in the mouth, rapid or labored breathing, and finally respiratory distress

Eschar (a layer of burned skin) will form at the site of injury. With time, the eschar will slough off and be replaced with epithelium (new skin) if the burn is partial thickness, or with granulation tissue if the burn is full thickness. Full thickness burns may eventually heal, particularly across the joints, by wound contracture. The best definitive treatment for large open wounds is skin grafting.

Treatment

Directed toward burns of 20% TBSA or greater, and those with inhalation injury. (For small burns, focus 7-18 on wound care.)

Primary

1. Stop the burning process. Decontaminate chemical burns at the scene. Remove any hot synthetic clothing. For patients with tar burns, immerse the injured areas in cold water until the hot tar has cooled down.
2. Protect the C-spine. Cervical injury is common following high-speed motor vehicle accidents, explosions, high-voltage electrical injury or falls/jumps.
3. Airway. Secure the airway. Prophylactically intubate patients with mild symptoms of airway obstruction (swelling of the face, upper airway or larynx) or smoke inhalation injury, and before a prolonged aeromedical or ground evacuation. See Procedure: Intubate a Patient
4. Breathing. Give 100% O2 by non-rebreather mask for burn, shock or carbon monoxide poisoning. Intubated patients can be bag-ventilated for prolonged periods (up to 12 hours) during evacuation.
5. Circulation. IV circulatory support: insert 2 large-bore cannulas through (in order of preference): unburned skin, eschar, cut-down or Intraosseous cannula. Start Lactated Ringer's (LR) at 500 cc/hr for adults or 250 cc/hr for children age 5-15. Do not give an initial fluid bolus (contraindicated in burn patients), unless the patient has low blood pressure or major mechanical trauma (i.e., bleeding). Secure the lines with suture:

tape does not stick well to burned skin. This IV fluid rate will need to be adjusted based on burn size and weight (see paragraph 8 below). Insert Foley catheter to monitor fluid output.

6. Disability. Neurological exam and treat neuro injuries. Even patients with massive injuries should initially be alert, unless they have received drugs, have sustained a head injury, are in shock, or have ingested a toxic substance (carbon monoxide, drugs, alcohol).

7. Exposure and environment. Keep the patient warm by all available means (aluminum combat casualty blanket, warm IV fluids, sleeping bag, etc.). Burn patients lose heat through the damaged skin, and severe hypothermia can result if the environment is not kept hot. Cool only the smallest burns. Never soak a burn patient in wet linens unless he also has heat stroke. Monitor core temperature at least hourly if possible.

8. Fluid Resuscitation. Carefully measure burn size and pre-burn weight, and estimate fluid resuscitation needs according to the formula below.

9. Do a careful secondary survey. Remove all the clothing, roll the patient to inspect the back, and remove all jewelry (especially rings, since fingers can swell causing damage beneath rings). Examine the corneas with fluorescein and Wood's lamp, looking for corneal defects in all patients with facial burns and those who complain of eye problems. Treat corneal abrasions with ophthalmic antibiotics such as **erythromycin** and **gentamicin**. Look for non-thermal trauma. Burns can make it more difficult to detect spinal or extremity fractures, or intra-abdominal injury. A diagnostic peritoneal lavage can be done through burned skin. Check the tympanic membranes for rupture in blast injuries.

10. Open fractures in burn patients are at high risk for developing osteomyelitis. Immobilize the fracture with splints. A plaster cast can be used over a burn, but should be immediately bivalved to permit wound care and to allow for post-burn swelling. Definitive care is external fixation.

11. Use frequent, low-dose IV narcotics (e.g., **morphine, fentanyl, methadone**) for pain control. Avoid IM narcotics. IV **ketamine** is useful for painful procedures. Give **Phenergan** 25 mg IV, IM, or by mouth to potentiate the effects of narcotics and treat nausea.

12. Place a nasogastric tube to prevent gastric ileus, vomiting and aspiration. To prevent stress ulceration of the stomach and duodenum, give 30 cc of **magnesium**- or **aluminum-containing antacids** q 2 hrs., preferably via nasogastric tube. Clamp the tube for 30 minutes after each dose, or give an IV H2-blocker such as **cimetidine**.

13. Immunize against tetanus as needed.

14. If the patient will be evacuated within 24 hrs. of injury, then no specific wound care of the burn is needed. Otherwise, cleanse the burns with an antimicrobial solution and daily shower. (Use normal saline or similar to cleanse the face.) In general, do not debride small (< 2 cm

diameter) blisters if they are

intact, but unroof them if they rupture, lie across major joints, or are large. If the burns are in the scalp,

shave the hair. Apply an antimicrobial burn cream such as **silver sulfadiazine (Silvadene, Flamazine,**

etc.) or **mafenide acetate (Sulfamylon)** bid. Following application, the wounds can be left open, but in

the field it is best to cover the wounds with sterile gauze dressings or clean linen. IV **ketamine** or

narcotics are useful for pain control during dressing changes. Alternate topical treatment: apply

7-19

Bacitracin to the face and to burn areas. If burn creams are not available, a 0.5 percent solution of

silver nitrate in water is also very effective. Apply this solution to a thick layer of gauze dressings at least

once every 6 hrs (must be kept moist). Do not put silver nitrate on the face (stains the corneas black).

Other options: any antibiotic ointment, **Betadine** ointment or even honey.

15. Do not use prophylactic IV or oral antibiotics. A centimeter of redness surrounding a burn wound is

common, and results from local inflammation rather than true infection. If redness spreads and other

symptoms of infection appear, the patient has cellulitis and needs anti-streptococcal antibiotics

(**penicillin, vancomycin,** or 1st generation cephalosporin). When effective burn creams are not used,

the patient may develop invasive gram-negative burn wound infection. Look for systemic signs of sepsis

and changes in the color and odor of the burn wound. This is a life-threatening problem- give aggressive

fluid resuscitation, and two broad-spectrum IV antipseudomonal antibiotics (**piperacillin, ticarcillin** or a

3rd generation cephalosporin; and an aminoglycoside).

16. Burn patients need more calories and protein. Supplement patients with burns over 30 % TBSA with

milkshakes or any similar high-calorie, high-protein food source.

17. Burn patients with deep burns across most or all of the anterior and lateral chest may develop a "chesteschar

syndrome" during the first 24 h post-burn. Full-thickness burned skin (leathery, tight, and inelastic)

may act like a straightjacket, inhibiting chest movement during inspiration or bag ventilation. Using a scalpel or electrocautery, cut through the eschar on the chest from mid-clavicular line to anterior axillary line down past the costal margin. Then, connect right and left across the epigastrium. Do this procedure immediately when it is needed.

18. Burn patients with circumferential deep burns of the extremities are at risk for an extremity eschar syndrome, in which swelling beneath the inelastic eschar causes gradual constriction of the blood vessels. This can result in nerve and muscle damage, and eventually life-threatening infection of dead muscle and/or limb loss. This syndrome is diagnosed by loss of distal pulses in a patient with deep (full-thickness or deep partial thickness) burns of an extremity. (Note also that low blood pressure due to severe shock may also cause loss of peripheral pulses in burn patients.) Treat with escharotomy: incise the tight, inelastic eschar with a scalpel or electrocautery. Place the incision in the mid-lateral and/or midmedial line of the extremity. Cut all the way through the skin, but no deeper into the subcutaneous fat than is necessary to release the tension. Low-dose IV narcotics or **ketamine** will help control pain. Check distal pulses after the procedure to make sure it was successful.

Chemical Injuries

1. Decontaminate the patient. Decontaminate at the site of injury as thoroughly as possible. Determine exactly what compound caused the injury. Following decontamination, treat in the same manner as thermal injuries.

2. Acids or bases: brush off any solid material, then flush with copious amounts of water for at least 30 minutes for acids, hours for bases. Test the skin with pH paper to determine when it is safe to stop decontamination. Never attempt to neutralize a chemical by applying a basic compound to an acid burn. Burns of the eyes should be continuously irrigated (can use IV line) at the inner canthus. Alkali burns of the eyes may require irrigation for 8-12 hours.

3. White phosphorus (WP): an incendiary compound that ignites on contact with air at 32°C (89.6°F). To prevent this, wounds containing WP fragments must be continuously immersed in water, saline solution, or similar liquid. Remove the fragments in an operating room and place them in a container of water. A Wood's lamp (UV light) can be used in a dark room to identify these fluorescent fragments.

4. Hydrofluoric acid (HF): HF absorption can cause deep tissue damage and can deplete circulating calcium and magnesium, resulting in lethal dysrhythmias. Topical application of **calcium gluconate** in a gel such as **Surgilube** will chelate the fluoride anion and prevent systemic absorption. This mixture can be placed inside a surgical glove for those patients with

HF hand burns.

5. Tar and asphalt. Hot tar and asphalt cause a deep thermal injury. Cool the injured areas in water. Then, apply white petrolatum (**Vaseline**, etc.), mineral oil, or vegetable oil to the area in order to dissolve and soften the material. Do not apply gasoline or other petroleum-based solvents.

Fluid Resuscitation

1. If LR is not available, you may use normal saline or alternate between normal saline and sodium bicarbonate solution (mix 2 1/2 50-meq ampules of **sodium bicarbonate** per liter of D5W to make a solution of 125 meq/L). If you give normal saline alone, you should also start D5W at the rate given below (1cc/kg/TBSA burned/24 h), because of the high sodium concentration in normal saline. You can also use 5% albumin (or fresh frozen plasma) during the first 24 hours post-burn in combination with crystalloid, according to a formula such as albumin (0.5 cc/kg/TBSA burned/24 h) plus LR or saline (1.5cc/kg/TBSA burned/24 h).

2. If unable to provide IV fluids, start oral resuscitation using the following oral formula: 1 liter of water, 1/4 tsp of salt, 1/4 tsp of sodium bicarbonate (if no bicarbonate, use total of 1/2 tsp salt), 2 tbsp. of sugar or honey and a little orange or lemon juice.

The following illustration shows the Rule of 9's

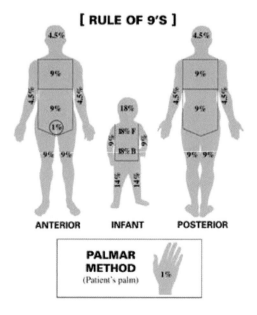

The following illustration shows where to make escharotomy incisions.

EMERGENCY ESCHAROTOMY

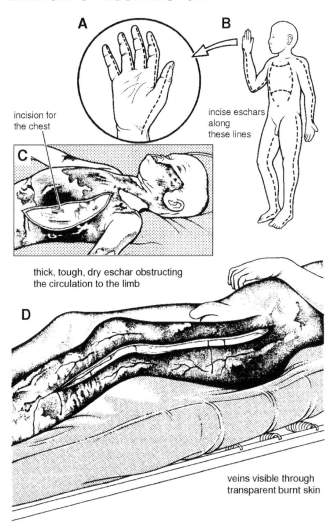

Parkland Burn Formula

The history of modern burn resuscitation can be traced back to observations made after large urban fires at the Rialto Theatre (New Haven, Conn) in 1921 and the Coconut Grove nightclub (Boston, Mass) in 1942. At the time, physicians noted that some patients with large burns survived the event but died from shock in the observation periods. Underhill and Moore identified the concept of thermal injury–induced intravascular fluid deficits in the 1930s and 1940s, and Evans soon followed with the earliest fluid resuscitation formulas in 1952. Up to that point, burns covering as little as 10-20% of total body surface area (TBSA) were associated with high rates of mortality. Through the 1970s, even a 30% TBSA burn was associated with nearly 100% mortality in older patients.

Over the next 50 years, advances in resuscitation further expanded these observations and led to numerous strategies to treat burn shock. The prognostic burn index (PBI), a crude estimate of mortality involving adding age + TBSA has steadily improved to the point that a PBI score of 90-100 (predicting near certain mortality) now demonstrates mortality rates of 50-70% in adult burns. Nearly 13,000 annual hospital admissions are attributable to burns, and almost a dozen deaths per day result from residential fires. Children younger than 5 years and adults older than 65 years have a mortality from burns that is 6 times the national average.

As the burn size approaches 15-20% total body surface area (TBSA), shock sets in if the patient does not undergo appropriate fluid resuscitation. The peak of this third-spacing occurs at some point 6-12 hours postburn as the capillary barrier begins to regain its integrity, hence the reduction in fluid requirements observed in resuscitation formulas around this point. At this point, the theoretic benefits of adjuvant colloid therapy during the resuscitation allow the careful downward titration of fluid administration to reduce the obligatory edema.

Other factors in burn edema include the heat-induced denaturing of collagen fibers in the interstitium, causing a physical expansion of the potential third space with a transient -20 to -30 mm Hg negative-pressure gradient favoring extravasation of fluid. In adults with burns approaching 25-30% TBSA, damage to cell membranes also occurs (observed in all forms of hypovolemic shock), which is associated with a decrease in transmembrane potential and the accumulation of intracellular sodium and water, with resultant swelling at the cellular level. Resuscitation is associated with a restoration of the transmembrane potential toward normal, but unlike hemorrhagic shock, this deficit is corrected only partially with burn shock and contributes to the multifactorial edema. Failure to aggressively treat the volume deficit properly leads to progressively decreasing membrane potential with eventual cell death.

The classic description of the burn wound and surrounding tissues is a system of several circumferential zones radiating from primarily burned tissues, as follows:

1. Zone of coagulation - A nonviable area of tissue at the epicenter of the burn
2. Zone of ischemia or stasis - Surrounding tissues (both deep and peripheral) to the coagulated areas, which are not devitalized initially but, due to microvascular insult, can progress irreversibly to necrosis over several days if not resuscitated properly
3. Zone of hyperemia - Peripheral tissues that undergo vasodilatory changes due to neighboring inflammatory mediator release but are not injured thermally and remain viable

The tissues in ischemic areas can potentially be salvaged by proper resuscitation in the initial stages and by proper burn wound excision and antimicrobial therapy in the convalescent period. Under resuscitation can convert this area into deep dermal or full-thickness burns in areas not initially injured to that extent. Reevaluation of these threatened areas over the first several days is used to determine when the first burn excision should be performed (i.e., when the depth of burn has become apparent and decisions about which areas are deep dermal or of full thickness are clear).

A new area of interest with immediate resuscitation is the use of sub atmospheric pressure dressings (e.g., the VAC by KCI) on affected areas. Animal models and early clinical work suggest that this treatment may limit the conversion of zones of hyperemia to zones of ischemia by removing edematous fluid and allowing salvage of areas that would otherwise need excision and grafting. Most useful in the authors' experience in this regard has been the use of circumferential upper extremity VAC dressings.

Historically, fluid management for burns has been as much an art as it has been a science; a fine line must be negotiated between an adequate resuscitation and one that is associated with the deleterious effects of fluid overload. Policies and practices have been highly individualized and can vary dramatically from institution to institution. However, the predominant teaching of the last quarter century has a pedigree derived from the influential publications involving regression analysis studies of resuscitative volumes in adult burn patients by Charles Baxter, MD, at Parkland Hospital at Southwestern University Medical Center (Dallas, TX) in the 1960s.

From these studies came the venerable Parkland formula, which advocated the guideline for total volume of the first 24 hours of resuscitation (with Ringer lactate [RL] solution) at approximately 4 mL/kg body weight per percentage burn TBSA. With this formula, half the volume is given in the first 8 hours post burn, with the remaining volume delivered over 16 hours. Multiple formulas exist with variations in both the volumes per weight suggested and the type or types of crystalloid or crystalloid-colloid combinations administered. To date, no single recommendation has been distinguished as the most successful approach.

The time-dependent variables for all of these formulas begin from the moment of injury, not from the time the patient is seen in the emergency department. A scenario that is not uncommon is a burn patient being transferred from an outlying hospital several hours after a burn and arriving in a severely under resuscitated or over resuscitated state. Calculations for the rate of fluid resuscitation should take this into account and reflect the decreased or increased starting IV fluid rate.

RL solution is a relatively isotonic crystalloid solution that is the key component of almost all resuscitative strategies, at least for the first 24-48 hours. It is preferable to isotonic sodium chloride solution (ie, normal saline [NS]) for large-volume resuscitations because its lower sodium concentration (130 mEq/L vs 154 mEq/L) and higher pH concentration (6.5 vs 5.0) are closer to physiologic levels. Another potential benefit of RL solution is the buffering effect of metabolized lactate on the associated metabolic acidosis. Plasmalyte is another crystalloid solution, the composition of which is even more closely physiologic than RL solution, and Plasmalyte is used in some centers as the initial crystalloid solution for large burns. However, the significant cost difference per unit, with an uncertain benefit, has limited its widespread use at many burn units.

Regardless of the resuscitation formula or strategy used, the first 24-48 hours require frequent adjustments. Calculated volumes from all of the formulas should be viewed as educated guesses of the appropriate fluid load. Blind adherence to a derived number can lead to significant over resuscitation or under resuscitation if not interpreted within the clinical context. Over resuscitation can be a major source of morbidity for burn patients and can result in increased pulmonary complications and escharotomies of the chest or extremities. In addition, not all burns require use of the Parkland formula for resuscitation. Promptly addressed adult burns of less than 15-20% TBSA without inhalation injury are usually not enough to initiate the systemic inflammatory response, and these patients can be rehydrated successfully primarily via the oral route with modest IV fluid supplementation.

An idea being advanced in some of the tertiary burn centers is to begin burn excision and wound closure *during* the resuscitation phase. The rationale for this strategy is to remove the devitalized tissue quickly to blunt the systemic inflammatory cascade.

Vital signs

Routine vital signs, such as blood pressure and heart rate, can be very difficult to interpret in patients with large burns. Catecholamine release during the hours after the burn can support blood pressures despite the extensive intravascular depletion that exists. The formation of edema in the extremities can limit the usefulness of noninvasive blood pressure measurements. Evaluation of arterial line pressures likewise is subject to error from peripheral vasospasm from the high-catecholamine state. Tachycardia, normally a clue to hypovolemia, can be secondary to pain and is also almost universally present from the adrenergic state. Following a trend in the gradual normalization of vital signs is thus much more useful than any single reading.

Vitamin C

A great deal of interest exists in using antioxidants as adjuncts to resuscitation to try to minimize oxidant-mediated contributions to the inflammatory cascade. In particular, mega dose vitamin C infusion during resuscitation has been studied at some length. Some animal models have demonstrated that infusion of vitamin C within 6 hours post burn can lower calculated resuscitation values by up to one half. Whether this phenomenon can be reproduced successfully in human subjects has not been clearly demonstrated.

Proponents have reached no consensus regarding the proper total dose. Some have adopted the strategy of placing up to 10 g in a liter of RL solution, infusing it at 100 mL/h (1 g/h vitamin C), and counting the volume as part of the resuscitation volume. Recently published data using an infusion of 66 mg/kg/h during the first 24 hours demonstrate a 45% decrease in the required fluid resuscitation in a small group of patients.

The safety of high-dose vitamin C has been established in humans, at least for the short-term, but this strategy is probably less safe in patients who are pregnant, those with renal failure, and those with a history of oxalate kidney stones.

End points for resuscitation

The end points for resuscitation are debatable, but hourly urine output is a well-established parameter for guiding fluid management. The rate of fluid administration should be titrated to a urine output of 0.5 mL/kg/h or approximately 30-50 mL/h in most adults and older children (>50 kg). In small children, the goal should be approximately 1 mL/kg/h (see Pediatric Resuscitation Issues). Failure to meet these goals should be addressed with gentle upward corrections in the rate of fluid administration by approximately 25%.

An important point is that periodically increasing the fluid rate is much more favorable than giving frequent boluses of fluid for low urine output. This results in transient elevations in hydrostatic pressure gradients that further increase the shift of fluids to the interstitium and worsen the edema. However, do not hesitate to administer a bolus to patients as appropriate early in the resuscitation for hypotensive shock. The urge to maintain urine output at rates greater than 30-50 mL/h should be avoided. Fluid overload in the critical hours of early burn management leads to unnecessary edema and pulmonary dysfunction. It can necessitate morbid escharotomies and extend the time required for ventilator support.

Several complicating factors exist with monitoring urine output as a guide for volume status and end organ perfusion. The presence of glycosuria can result in an osmotic diuresis and can lead to artificially elevated urine output values. Performing a urinalysis at some point during the first 8 hours can be prudent, especially for patients with larger burns, to screen for this potentially serious overestimation of the intravascular volume. In addition, older patients with long-standing diuretic use may be dependent on diuretics and may not be able to maintain a desired urine output despite what appears to be an adequate resuscitation volume. Swan-Ganz catheter placement is an important adjunct in the decision-making process in this group of patients regarding fluid replacement and possible diuretic use.

Other physiologic parameters that reflect the adequacy of resuscitation include an improving base deficit and the maintenance of the cardiac index in those in whom invasive monitors are placed. Because of several factors, such as pulmonary vasoconstriction, the same interpretive problems are true for central venous pressure or pulmonary capillary wedge pressure measurements. Swan-Ganz catheters should not be used routinely but may have some role in geriatric patients and those with poor underlying cardiac function.

Again, the overall clinical response and general trends in these numbers are much more useful for adjusting fluid administration or chemotherapy to support cardiac function than values from isolated measurements. Catheter-based resuscitation tends to deliver higher-based volumes then the traditional methods but has not demonstrated an improvement in morbidity or mortality. Research indicates that increased crystalloid cannot restore cardiac preload to baseline during the period of burn shock.

Certain patient populations frequently require resuscitation volumes that are higher than those calculated. Patients with inhalation injuries are perhaps the most studied subset, with required volumes sometimes as much as 30-40% higher (close to 5.7 mL/kg per percentage) than predicted by the Parkland formula for adequate resuscitation. Delays in initiating resuscitation promptly have also been shown to increase fluid requirements by as much as 30%, presumably by permitting the occurrence of an increased inflammatory cascade. Patients on home diuretic therapy frequently have preexisting free-water deficits in addition to burn shock. The presence of an escharotomy or fasciotomy can substantially increase free water loss from the wound, and this must be replaced. Patients with electrical burns, often associated with large and underappreciated tissue insult, likewise require large-volume fluid resuscitations.

Do not forget that burn patients are trauma patients and frequently arrive with a poor history of the events surrounding the accident. An unexpected high volume requirement should therefore prompt a very close examination for missed associated injuries. A strategy that has been used with some success for refractory burn shock has been investigated by researchers at the University of Cincinnati and involves plasma exchange. Appropriate candidates for this innovative technique include those with more than twice the calculated fluid requirements despite hypertonic saline infusion.

Table 2. Resuscitation Formulas

Formula	Fluid in First 24 Hours	Crystalloid in Second 24-Hours	Colloid in Second 24-Hours
Parkland	RL at 4 mL/kg per percentage burn	20-60% estimated plasma volume	Titrated to urinary output of 30 mL/h
Evans	NS at 1 mL/kg per percentage burn, 2000 mL D5W*, and colloid	50% of first 24-hour volume plus 2000 mL	50% of first 24-hour volume

	at 1 mL/kg per percentage burn	D5W	
Slater	RL at 2 L/24 h plus fresh frozen plasma at 75 mL/kg/24 h		
Brooke	RL at 1.5 mL/kg per percentage burn, colloid at 0.5 mL/kg per percentage burn, and 2000 mL D5W	50% of first 24-hour volume plus 2000 mL D5W	50% of first 24-hour volume
Modified Brooke	RL at 2 mL/kg per percentage burn		
Metro Health (Cleveland)	RL solution with 50 mEq sodium bicarbonate per liter at 4 mL/kg per percentage burn	Half NS titrated to urine output	1 U fresh frozen plasma for each liter of half NS used plus D5W as needed for hypoglycemia
Monafo hypertonic Demling	250 mEq/L saline titrated to urine output at 30 mL/h, dextran 40 in NS at 2 mL/kg/h for 8 hours, RL titrated to urine output at 30 mL/h, and fresh frozen plasma 0.5 mL/h for 18 hours beginning 8 hours post burn	One-third NS titrated to urine output	
*D5W is dextrose 5% in water solution			

Due to the high morbidity associated with high-volume resuscitations, an interest exists in using various colloid solutions to both decrease edema and volume requirements and blunt the myocardial depression phenomena observed with large burns. An important consideration for adding colloid in the first 24 hours is the loss of capillary integrity during early burn shock. This process occurs early and is present for 8-24 hours depending on which authority is referenced. A strategy for testing whether the capillary leak has begun to resolve involves substituting an equal volume of albumin solution for RL solution. An increase in urine output suggests that at least some of the leak has resolved and that the further introduction of colloid can help decrease the fluid load.

Albumin is the plasma protein that most contributes to intravascular oncotic pressure. When administered intravenously as a 5% solution from pooled plasma product, approximately half the volume remains intravascularly, as opposed to 20-30% of crystalloid solutions. Alternatively, some centers prefer using fresh frozen plasma over using albumin because of the theoretic advantage of replacing the whole range of plasma proteins that are lost rather than just the albumin fraction. Guidelines for this infusion have been reported as 0.5-1 mL/kg per percentage burn during the first 24 hours, beginning 8-10 hours postburn as an adjuvant to RL solution resuscitation.

Dextran is a solution of polymerized, high molecular weight glucose chains with almost twice the oncotic pressure of albumin. An increase in microcirculatory flow is also produced by reducing erythrocyte aggregation. Proponents of dextran point to the reduction of edema in nonburned tissues as justification for its use. The edema-reducing properties are maintained for as long as the infusion is continued, but upon withdrawal and subsequent metabolism of the glucose, rapid loss of fluid occurs back into the interstitium if the capillary leak is still present. Demling and others have used dextran 40 successfully in the early postburn period (first 8 h) at 2 mL/kg/h along with RL solution before switching to some albumin or fresh frozen plasma plus RL solution combination for the second 18-hour phase.

Hypertonic saline solutions, ranging in concentration from 180-300 mEq sodium per liter, have many theoretic benefits. These benefits are achieved by the reduction in volume requirements by mobilizing intracellular fluid into the vascular space by the increased osmotic gradient. The intracellular depletion of water that results is a debated concern, but it appears to be well tolerated. Close monitoring of serum sodium levels is mandatory, and serum sodium levels should not be allowed to increase to greater than 160 mEq/dL.

As a compromise strategy to limit the risk of hypernatremia and sodium retention, some institutions use RL solution with 50 mEq amps of sodium bicarbonate per bag, for a fluid approaching 180 mEq sodium per liter during the initial 8 hours of the resuscitation, rather than using the more concentrated saline solutions. Then, after the first 8 hours, the fluid is changed to RL solution to complete the resuscitation. Hypertonic saline management must be titrated closely to both urine output and serum sodium checks and probably should not be used routinely outside of tertiary burn centers.

The safety and benefits of hypertonic saline resuscitation extend to both the pediatric and geriatric populations, but using solutions at the lower end of tonicity is probably safer. The greatest benefit may ultimately be for those patients with the most limited cardiopulmonary reserves, those with inhalation injury, and those with larger burns approaching 40% or more.

Exactly when or whether to add colloid to resuscitation fluids is a confusing issue. As mentioned previously, most of the mainstream burn formulas add colloid during the resuscitation, at least in the second 24-hour period. However, what must be recognized is that despite a general consensus that colloid use is both beneficial and appropriate, especially in burns greater than 40% TBSA, demonstrating improved outcomes in morbidity or mortality has been difficult. In fact, some studies have demonstrated harmful effects secondary to increased pulmonary edema and some evidence of renal dysfunction as manifested by a decreased glomerular filtration rate. For smaller burns (ie, 20-40% without inhalation injury), expectant management with RL solution titrated to urine output is a safe and well-tested strategy.

The patients who benefit the most from lower-volume resuscitations aided by colloid are those with larger burns (>40%), those with preexisting heart disease, geriatric patients, and those with burns with associated inhalation injuries

At 24-30 hours after the insult, the patient should be resuscitated adequately, with near complete resolution of the transcapillary leak with fluid requirements. At this point, some authorities recommend a change in fluid management from RL solution to a combination fluid infusion involving albumin and D5W. The rational for this is the massive protein losses that have occurred from the burn wound during the first 24 hours. Replacing this deficit with a steady infusion of 5% or 25% albumin solution can serve to maintain a serum albumin concentration greater than 2, which can help reduce tissue edema and improve gut function. Associated insensible losses of free water from the injured skin barrier can be met by replacing the deficit with an electrolyte-free fluid such as D5W solution, which also serves to restore the extracellular space to an isotonic state, especially if hypertonic solutions were used during the resuscitation.

The formula for the estimate for 5% albumin infusion is as follows:
0.5 mL/kg per percentage burn = mL albumin for 24 hours

The formula for the free water estimate is as follows:

(25 + percentage burn) X BSA (m^2) = mL/h of free water required
The US Army Institute of Surgical Research uses a similar approach but stratifies the albumin calculations by the estimated TBSA of the burn. For burns of 30-50%, they use 0.3 mL/kg per percentage burn; for burns of 50-70%, 0.4 mL/kg per percentage burn is used; and for burns of 70% and greater, they use 0.5 mL/kg per percentage burn.

A potential pitfall is iatrogenic hypernatremia as a result of titrating a sodium-rich albumin solution. Serum sodium levels should be checked at least once a day. The relative rate of albumin is titrated to adequate urine output with close monitoring of the serum sodium level. As the serum sodium level rises to unacceptable levels, simply increasing the D5W solution infusion rate corrects it toward normal or vice versa.

The most important thing to recognize with all the discussion regarding fluid management is that many different techniques have proven successful. Replacing the volume deficit to support tissue perfusion and correct the metabolic acidosis can be achieved with multiple fluid types and has been the rationale for treatment for nearly 70 years. Changes to this basic tenet have only come at the periphery. Real progress in the understanding of the very complex associated pathophysiology of burn shock is reflected in the use of newer products to supplement crystalloid resuscitation. Further advances will obviously come from optimizing the timing of the colloid and hypertonic administration and from research into blunting the underlying mediators of burn shock.

Pediatric Resuscitation Issues

Since the recognition of the phenomenon of burn shock, significant progress has been made in the survival rates of pediatric and juvenile patients. Currently, patients with all but the largest TBSA injuries can be expected to survive when treated promptly.

Several very important conceptual differences exist in pediatric burn resuscitation. Intravenous fluid resuscitations are usually required for patients with smaller burns (in the range of 10-20%). Venous access in small children may be a difficult issue, and a saphenous vein cutdown or an interosseous line is an acceptable alternative in the short term.

Children have proportionally larger BSAs than adults; TBSA burns must be estimated using pediatric modifications to Lund-Browder tables, which demonstrate the relatively larger head and small thigh. This results in higher weight-based calculations for resection volume (nearly 6 mL/kg per percentage burn) and has led some to advocate a BSA-based resuscitation in addition to the infusion of a maintenance requirement as described by the Galveston Shriners Hospital pediatric formula. Other centers, such as the Shriners Burn Institute in Cincinnati, Ohio, simply use the Parkland formula with the addition of a maintenance rate.

Recommended end points are also higher in children, with urine output closer to 1 mL/kg/h being a more appropriate goal. Children approaching 50 kg are probably better served by adult resuscitation parameters (30-50 mL/h urine output) and calculations. Another concern with this population is the modest hepatic glycogen reserves, which can be exhausted quickly and sometimes require the change from RL solution to dextrose 5% in RL solution to prevent life-threatening hypoglycemia. For this reason, AccuChecks every 4-6 hours should be routine during the hypermetabolic state, especially for patients with larger burns.

Pediatric resuscitation protocols are based on the following formula (H is height [cm], W is weight [kg]):
BSA = [87 (H + W) - 2600] / 10,000

Pediatric resuscitation protocols are as follows:

- Shriners Burn Institute (Cincinnati) - 4 mL/kg per percentage burn plus 1500 mL/m² BSA
    - First 8 hours - RL solution with 50 mEq sodium bicarbonate per liter
    - Second 8 hours - RL solution
    - Third 8 hours - RL solution plus 12.5 g of 25% albumin solution per liter
- Galveston Shriners Hospital - 5000 mL/m² TBSA burn plus 2000 mL/m²BSA, using RL solution plus 12.5 g 25% albumin per liter plus D5W solution as needed for hypoglycemia.

The most important thing to remember regarding fluid management is that many different techniques have proven successful. Replacing the volume deficit to support tissue perfusion and correct the metabolic acidosis can be achieved with multiple fluid types and has been the rationale for treatment for nearly 70 years.

Changes to this basic tenet have only come at the periphery. Real progress in the understanding of the very complex associated pathophysiology of burn shock is reflected in the use of newer products to supplement crystalloid resuscitation.

According to retrospective analysis, most important predictors of mortality are the size of burn, age of patient, and worst base deficit in the first 24 hours. Further advances will obviously come from optimizing the timing of colloid and hypertonic fluid administration and from research into blunting the underlying mediators of burn shock.

9 CONCLUSION

I have been fortunate (or unfortunate) enough to have been able to use every technique described in this book on more than one occasion. The thing about Advanced First Aid you have to remember is that you can do far more harm than good.

One axiom you need to live by is, ***"When in doubt, Don't do it!"*** If you aren't sure if your patient has a tension pneumothorax, don't dart their chest. If you aren't sure if they need stiches, don't put them in. Use less invasive measures first, ***ALWAYS***. Don't jump right into doing a surgical cricothyrotomy when a nasal airway will do the job.

Remember the 3 R's when it comes to performing any advanced technique.

- Right Patient- Make sure your patient NEEDS the procedure you are about to perform
- Right Procedure- Make sure you are using the LEAST invasive procedure to correct the problem
- Right Place- Make sure you are placing that chest tube, airway, IV, etc. in the right location

And if you are giving ANY MEDICATION at all to a patient here are a three more R's you need to remember to avoid killing your patient.

- Right Medication- Make sure you are giving the right medication for the problem you are trying to correct (You don't want to

give your Aunt Edna her high blood pressure medication when her blood pressure is 80/30 because she is hypovolemic for example)
- Right Dose- You want to make sure that you are giving the right dosage of any given medication (Don't give a 4 year old child the adult dose of Tylenol just because that is all you have and they have a high fever. Do the math and figure out how to cut the pill up so they get the proper dose)
- Right Route- You need to make sure you are giving medication the way it is meant to be given. If you are supposed to inject it into a muscle don't give it through an IV, if you are supposed to give it by mouth don't crush it up and make it so you can give it by injection. Giving medication by any route except as it is supposed to given can kill your patient.

Another thing you have to do is keep calm! Getting overly excited and letting it show does a couple of things:

- It will stress your patient out. They have enough to worry about without having to wonder if you are going to do the right thing and save their life. By remaining calm you will project confidence in your skills and your ability
- It will cause "Tunnel Vision", I have seen more medics (and a few doctors) than I can count completely miss a serious injury because they got excited at all the blood gushing from a very superficial scalp wound.
- It will project a sense that you don't know what the hell you are doing to the rest of your team causing them to focus on you and what you are doing and not on what they should be doing, pulling security or shooting back!

I can't stress enough that the information contained in this book **CAN KILL** if not used correctly and as such I, Vanguard Survival, LLC, nor Vanguard Survival Press are responsible for any injury, disability, or death that results from you using any of the techniques in this book, you are using any/all of the information presented in this book **AT YOUR OWN RISK** and without any warranty from the author or Vanguard Survival, LLC, Vanguard Survival Press, our agents, or assigns.

BIBLIOGRAPHY

National Association of Emergency Medical Technicians. *Pre-Hospital Trauma Life Support , Military Edition.* Elsevier Science Health Science Division. 2014. Print

National Association of Emergency Medical Technicians. *Pre-Hospital Trauma Life Support 8th Edition.* Elsevier/ Mosby 2013. Print

Pal, Neelu MD. *Emergency Escharotomy.* emedicine.medscape.com. June 2014

Grey, Henry. *Anatomy of the Human Body.* Lea & Febiger, 1918. Print

Special Operations Command. *Special Operation Medical Handbook.* Defense Department. 2013. Print

Special Operations Command. *Ranger Medical Handbook 4th Edition.* Defense Department. 2012. Print

Moses, Scott MD. *Fluid Resuscitation in Trauma.* www.fpnotebook.com. May 2014

Giddings. F. *Surgical Knots and Suturing Techniques 4th Edition.* Giddings Studio Publishing. 2013. Print

Stewart, Charles E. *Advanced Airway Management*. Brady. 2002. Print

Khan, Huma MD; Meyers, Arlen D MD, MBA. *Cricothyroidotomy*. emedicine.medscape.com. May 2014

Laws, D MD. *BTS Guidelines for the Insertion of a Chest Drain*. Thorax.bmj.com. June 2014

American College of Surgeons Committee on Trauma. *Thoracic trauma. Advanced Trauma Life Support program for physicians: Instructor manual*. Chicago: American College of Surgeons, 1993.

Bledsoe, Bryan E.; Porter, Robert S.; Cherry, Richard A. *Paramedic Care: Principles & Practice, Volume 3: Patient Assessment, 4th Edition*. Prentice Hall. 2012

Campbell, John E. *BTLS: Basic Trauma Life Support*. Brady Prentice Hall. 2011. Print

American Heart Association. *Advanced Cardiovascular Life Support (ACLS) for Healthcare Providers*. AHA. 2012. Print

Irion, Glenn. *Comprehensive Wound Management*. SLACK Incorporated. 2010. Print

Hauser, Alan R. *Antibiotic Basics for Clinicians: Choosing the Right Antibacterial Agent*. Lippincott Williams & Wilkins. 2007. Print

Sussman, Carrie; Bates-Jensen, Barbara M. *Wound Care: A Collaborative Practice Manual for Physical Therapists and Nurses*. Aspen Publishers. 2008. Print

Blantyre, Malawi. *Effects of honey and sugar dressings on wound healing*. National Institutes of Health. 2007. Print

Herndon, David N. *Total Burn Care 4th Edition*. Elsevier Health Sciences. 2012. Print

ABOUT THE AUTHOR

Tom served in the US Army for over 10 years, after leaving the service Tom pursued a career as a paramedic eventually becoming a Tactical Medic for the local police department SWAT team. Shortly after 9/11 Tom found himself in Afghanistan.

In 2005 Tom was wounded and again found himself a civilian, after recovering from his wounds Tom went to work as a civilian contractor first as a medic and eventually as a Team Leader on convoy escort missions in Afghanistan, Iraq, and Africa.

In 2007 Tom returned to the states and moved to Key West where he managed the largest bar on the island. In 2009 Tom married his wife Tiffany and in 2011 Tom and his family moved back to Colorado where, with the encouragement of his wife and friends Tom started Vanguard Survival, LLC so he could provide real world based survival and weapons training.

This is Tom's third book on survival related topics for Vanguard Survival Press.

Tom lives with his wife, Tiffany, 5 kids, 3 dogs, 3 spastic cats, 2 ferrets, a handful of mice, and a ball python

Made in the USA
Lexington, KY
30 October 2015